# Autophagy

*Discover How to Cleanse your Body, Activate The Metabolism,and Improve your Life with the Intermittent Fasting*

# Disclaimer Warning:

All of the content and information contained within the book are to be used for entertainment, educational, or personal use only. Every effort has been made to provide the most updated, true, dependable, and comprehensive information possible. There are no warranties implied or acknowledged here whatsoever. Several different sources were used to help produce the information within the book. Do not attempt to use any of the techniques or methods mentioned in this book without first getting a professional consultation from a licensed expert.

By reading the material contained within the book, you acknowledge that no professional, health/medical, legal, or financial advice or consultation is being offered by the author or publisher. You also agree never to hold the author liable for any losses that you've suffered, whether indirectly or directly, as a result of utilizing the content published within the book, including inaccuracies, omissions, errors, and other unintentional mistakes.

# Table of Contents

# INTRODUCTION

Congratulations on downloading *Autophagy:* *Discover How to Cleanse your Body, Activate the Metabolism, and Improve Your Life with the Intermittent Fasting*, and thank you for doing so. With increasing industrialization and increased productivity, the diet of humans has changed. Processed and unhealthy foods are becoming more affordable compared to natural healthier foods. This has contributed to the increasing cases of overweight and obesity across the world, with millions of people succumbing to weight-related conditions such as high blood pressure, obesity, and diabetes. With the rising overweight cases, many people have turned to diets, which they believe can help them lose weight. However, most people have experienced failure in such strategies, which have continuously caused depression and more desperation for better options. By downloading this book, you have taken the first step towards learning how to lose weight naturally through autophagy. The information that you find in the following chapters is very important as it will help you to take control of your body weight as well as increase your chances of preventing heart-related diseases such as stroke and high blood pressure.

To that end, this book provides an in-depth overview of autophagy and its role in weight loss. The book highlights the definition of autophagy, including the history and development of autophagy and its application in weight loss. It then covers the ways through which autophagy aids in weight loss. People who suffer from overweight and frequent gaining of weight are more likely to have poor relationships with food. Thus, this book will comprehensively address the strategies through which one can improve their weight loss journey while still having a positive relationship with food. An interesting concept covered in this book is the intermittent fasting; the final chapter covers the different types of intermittent fasting and their correlation with autophagy. With this knowledge, you will be able to learn how to manage your weight.

I have included a lot of useful information regarding hypnotherapy and its role in weight loss. I hope you enjoy reading!

Thanks very much for choosing this book, make sure to leave a short review on Amazon ifYou like it. I'm very interesting to see Your comments.

# CHAPTER:-1

## INTRODUCTION TO AUTOPHAGY

Just as cells ought to manufacture vital components for optimal functioning, so must they break down damaged, dismissed, or unnecessary organelles and any other cellular components. For cells to maintain this delicate balance, they make use of an essential degradative pathway called autophagy.

Autophagy is your body's way of cleaning out any damaged cells to generate newer, healthier cells. "Auto" means self while "phagy" means eat, so literally, autophagy is the process through which your body consumes itself. The old cells are broken down and discarded or recycled to make newer healthier cells. The idea behind autophagy is that when you deprive your body of external sources of food, your body will begin to eat itself, and in the process, it destroys and recycle its damaged cell bit and protein. It will then regenerate new and much healthier cells that can withstand stress and photogenic invasion. Autophagy plays a crucial role in protecting against diseases such as cancer and dementia, among many others.

Although autophagy occurs regularly in your body, subjecting your body to food deprivation through fasting and any other form of stress such as intense workouts appears to accelerate it further to achieve a type of cleansing overdrive.

Studies have determined that increased levels of autophagy in people could be responsible for increased longevity. It has also been established that autophagy helps fight infectious disease and regulate your body's inflammation as well as boosting your immune system.

But perhaps, it is the link between and cancer that has interested researcher's world over. The researchers are keen on establishing how fasting-induced autophagy interacts with cancerous cells. They believe that autophagy induced through fasting confuses and weakens the cancerous cells, and once other traditional drugs are added, the cells suffer instant death. In this way, researchers believe that autophagy acts as a tumor suppressor.

Moreover, autophagy has a lot of health benefits to your body. It is an evolutionary process through which your body self-preserve itself by removing any dysfunctional cells and recycling parts of them for cellular repair and cleaning. One of the critical roles of autophagy is to remove any debris in your body for your body to regulate back and achieve its optimal functioning.

Autophagy is also essential in promoting your body's survival and adaptation as a response to a variety of stressors and toxins, which are accumulated in your cells.

## The Process of Autophagy

Autophagy is induced by nutrient limitation as well as cellular stress. This governs the degradation of a significant number of long-lived proteins making up the cells, protein aggregates as well as other organelles in your body. It enables cells to withstand stress from the external environment, for example, nutrients deprivation as well as internal stress such as the accumulation of damaged organelles and any pathogen invasion. When you starve yourself, you automatically induce autophagy by degrading superfluous intracellular components and reusing the breakdown products, thus enabling you to survive periods of scarce nutrients.

Autophagy can also be induced during specific developmental states as a response to various hormonal imbalance.

## The Origin of Autophagy

Keith R. Ports, and his student, Thomas Ashford, first discovered Autophagy in the year 1962 at the Rockefeller Institute. They observed an increase in the number of lysosomes when they added glucagon to lab rat cells, which they were studying. They also noted that displaced lysosomes at the center of the cell had traces of cell organelles. The critical cell organelles were mitochondria. They coined the name autolysis for this process.

Inspired by this discovery, de Duve came up with the name autophagy in 1963 to describe the process through which glycogen induces cell degradation in your liver. Christian de Duve was a Belgium Biochemist instrumental in various biochemical research breakthroughs. Together with his student Russell Deter, he established that lysosomes are responsible for the glucagon inducing Autophagy.

In the early 90s, several scientists carried out extensive research, which discovered Autophagy related genes by making use of the budding yeast. Some of the key researchers included Ohsumi Yoshinori and his counterpart Michael Thumm. These two researchers are responsible for the discovery of starvation-induced autophagy, which is non-selective across all mammals.

At the turn of the 21st century, the area of Autophagy experienced some accelerated growth. Scientists were keen on establishing the functions and the roles of Autophagy in human health and diseases.

In 1999, a group of scientists known as the Beth Levine group made a landmark discovery. They established a connection between autophagy and cancer. From then, the scientist has concentrated their attention and tools to dissect the roles that autophagy plays in the suppression of the cancerous cells.

In the year 2003, a significant conference on autophagy was held in the city of Waterville. This conference, which was christened Gordon research conference aimed at bringing all autophagy researchers together for them to share their experiences in this field. This conference was closely followed by the establishment and the launching of a scientific journal called *Autophagy i*n the year 2005. This journal sought to provide all essential data on autophagy, which the scientists could use as a reference point.

In 2007, the first Keystone Conference focusing on the development of autophagy was held in Monterey. The conference sought to find ways through which researchers could further accelerate their work with the hope of finding a sustainable solution to cancer through autophagy.

In 2008, a scientist named Carol Mercer successfully created a BHMT fusion protein, which gave credence to the belief that fasting triggers Autophagy in mammals. The research showed that when a cell is starved of its nutrients, it automatically leads to the fragmentation in the cell lines. BHMT is a metabolic enzyme that is used to determine autophagy flux in your cells.

And in 2016, a Japanese biologist called Yoshinori Ohsumi received a Nobel prize for his discoveries and research on autophagy. He established the mechanisms underlying Autophagy.

Autophagy continues to gain more attention and interest from researchers who are keen on carrying out further studies to develop the other impacts it has on your health. Various researchers agree that there is much that is needed to learn about autophagy and how best one can encourage it to benefit most from the process. It is also a universal agreement with the researchers that the field is still entirely new, and much of the lingering questions on autophagy remain mostly unanswered.

## Benefits of Autophagy

It may sound somewhat awkward if you are told you stand to benefit when your body eats itself. But this is true. Self-eating by your body could be a fountain of renewed youthfulness. Autophagy enables your cells to go into a mode through which they repair any damage and self-heal themselves. The body activates the healing mode when it needs to save energy or fight an infection or when it wants to repair any worn-out cells. The following are some of the critical benefits of autophagy that you should be aware of:

## Autophagy can save your life

It has been scientifically proven that self-eating autophagy mechanisms are actually designed to preserve your life. Whenever you are exposed to extreme stress or infection and starvation, your body automatically triggers the process of Autophagy to repair the damage and prevent the development of the disease-causing pathogens. The method of autophagy ensures the intruding pathogens are starved of glucose, thus reducing inflammation and boosting your immune system to tackle the infectious intruder.

This way, autophagy in animals plays a central role in the human immune system's capability to fight illnesses and reduce the risk of diseases such as cancer.

## Autophagy is key to quality life and increased life span

Recent studies reveal that autophagy helps to slow and reverse your aging process. The studies reveal that autophagy enables cells to recycle the damaged parts and remove unwanted toxic material in a self-cleansing process. When the cells repair themselves, they tend to function better and behave like new younger cells. Toxins in your body are responsible for damage and aging. Thus, autophagy can significantly help you to reverse the effects of aging, making you look younger once again. Studies on lab mice have also established that autophagy is critical in extending your lifespan. A group of mice was starved to achieve the state of autophagy, and researchers noted that these mice were able to live longer than their peers who ate usually.

## Autophagy aids your metabolism process

The process of autophagy involves the taking out of unwanted cell parts and replacement of the cell parts such as mitochondria. Mitochondria acts as your cellular engines. Their primary function is to burn fat to make ATP. ATP is responsible for your body's energy needs. Mitochondria accumulate a lot of trash during its normal functioning. This trash can easily damage your cells. When these trashes are broken down and gotten rid of by autophagy your cells are saved of further damage through wear and tear.

Autophagy also aids your cells to function efficiently in the burning of fuel and production of protein. They make your cells to be new, healthy, and efficient in their work.

## Autophagy reduces your risk of getting neurodegenerative diseases.

When proteins in or around your cells are misfolded, they tend to stop working well. Autophagy is vital in helping cells to clean up the proteins that are not functioning well. They also help in clearing up these proteins and prevent further accumulation. A good example is an amyloid in Alzheimer's disease. Autophagy is responsible for the removal of dysfunctional amyloid. Another example is the removal of a-synuclein in Parkinson's disease by the process of autophagy.

## Autophagy helped in the regulation of inflammation

Autophagy help regulates or prevents inflammation

in your body by boosting your body's immune response to your needs. When an invader is detected in your body, autophagy increases the inflammation. The increase in inflammation triggers your immune system to attack the intruder. But during healthy times, autophagy decreases the inflammation in your body by suppressing the signals that trigger it.

## Autophagy helps your body to fight infectious diseases

Autophagy contributes to trigger an immune response whenever your body is under attack from diseases carrying pathogens. Besides, the process of autophagy can remove disease-causing microbes directly from inside the infected cells. For example, autophagy can remove microbes from mycobacterium tuberculosis or in viruses such as HIV.

Besides, autophagy can also get rid of toxins that are left behind by the infections in your cells. This process is essential in the prevention of foodborne diseases.

## Autophagy improves the performance of your muscles

After workouts, your muscles tend to tear and wear and would need repair or replacement. Most of the damage is caused by too much energy which is needed by your muscles whenever you are engaging in exercises. Your muscle cells can repair the damage by undergoing autophagy to reduce the energy demand when muscles are in use in order to degrade the damaged parts and maintain the balance of energy needed so as to reduce the risk of damage in the future.

## Autophagy can prevent the onset of cancer

Autophagy plays an essential role in the suppression of cancer-causing processes such as chronic inflammation. It also suppresses pro-cancer processes such as genome instability as well as the DNA damage response. When cancerous cells progress, it seeks an alternative source of fuel, and as a result, it activates the process of autophagy.

## Autophagy improves your digestive system

Much work is done by the cells lining up your gastrointestinal tract, and as such, they endure much wear and tear. When your body turns to autophagy, your tract cells are repaired and restored to function optimally. Autophagy also helps the cells to rid themselves of the unwanted junk and activate the immune system whenever necessary.

## Autophagy improves your skin health

Your skin cells take in a lot of damage due to exposure to chemicals, heat, cold, and other weather veracities. When the skin cells accumulate a lot of waste and toxins, they age substantially. Autophagy can help regenerate new skin cells that will help your skin glow.

## The negative side of Autophagy

Although autophagy controls inflammation, studies have established that some bacteria like Brucellas, Coxiella and Lyme use autophagy to recreate and replicate themselves.

This cell replicating process is also dominant in some cancer-causing cells. Self-eating can also enhance tumor cell's fitness against environmental stressors, making them more resilient to starvation and chemotherapy. It is, therefore, wise to use autophagy to prevent cancer but not as a treatment.

In conclusion, while autophagy eliminates some pathogens and viruses, some of these pathogens and viruses hijack the process of autophagy to replicate themselves.

# CHAPTER:-2

## HOW AUTOPHAGY WORKS

By now, the term autophagy is quite familiar to you. You are also aware of the origin and development, as well as the key benefits of autophagy to your overall health. In this chapter, we will strive to understand how autophagy works in your body.

First, it is essential to note that your cells accumulate a lot of dead organelles over time. They also accumulate damaged proteins as well as oxidized particles. The accumulation of these debris clogs and affects your body's inner workings.

When your body's optimal working conditions are affected by the accumulation of the unwanted debris, your aging process is accelerated substantially. Your risk of getting exposure to diseases such as cancer and other age-related disorders such as dementia is also increased significantly.

Your body then develops a unique way of getting rid of the damaged, diseased, or worn-out cells and cell parts to enable crucial cells such as the brain cells to last for a lifetime. This unique way is what is called autophagy and is critical in empowering your body to naturally defend itself against any invasion by disease-causing pathogens.

## How Autophagy Works

For you to understand better how autophagy works in your body, we are going to use two analogies:

**Analogy 1:**In the first analogy, we are going to take your body as a busy kitchen. After you have made your food, you usually keep your kitchen clean by getting rid of any leftovers and any accumulated dirt. The cleaning helps to maintain your kitchen in pristine conditions and makes it conducive for the next meal preparation. You also recycle any food left for use in the subsequent day. This is how autophagy works in your body. It gets rid of any worn-out cells and accumulated debris. It then regenerates new cells which can work better and defend your body against any disease infections.

**Analogy 2:** We will use the same kitchen scenario, but because of old age, you can't perform your duties of cleaning the kitchen well. So, after cooking, you leave all the dirt behind. They deposit on the counter, and over time, the toxic waste undergoes food fermentation. This results in nasty smells as the food remnants undergo decomposition. Your kitchen becomes a haven of toxins, pollutants, and germs. This is what happens in your body in the absence of autophagy.

The process of autophagy in your body takes place subconsciously and silently behind the scenes as it goes about its maintenance business. However, the process is put into high gear during the periods of extreme stress. This is the natural way through which your response against stress agents such as famine or infections. Activating autophagy in your body, therefore, results in the slowing of the aging process. It also reduces your body's inflammation rates to boost your immune system.

## Explanation of Autophagy Process: The Scientific Way

A recent study conducted by Newcastle University reveals that humans can live longer because of the adaptations in a protein commonly known as p62. P62 helps you to respond better when exposed to any biological stressors. The process of autophagy induces the p62 protein.

The P62 protein activates autophagy to start cleansing once it senses metabolic by-products that cause damage in your body. These by-products are scientifically referred to as reactive oxygen species or ROS. The p62 proteins work by removing all damaged and unwanted parts in your cell, enabling you to be better equipped to fight any biological stress. This process is critical for making you look younger and healthier.

The researchers also established that this process is unique to humans. They used fruit flies to understand the process of autophagy in humans. In their studies, the fruit flies failed to kick start the process of autophagy, so the researches sought an explanation for this failure. It was established that the part of the human p62 protein enables your body to sense ROS.

They then created genetically modified flies using humanized p62 protein. The result was that the humanized flies were able to survive for long periods when exposed to stressful conditions as compared to their peers. They concluded that humans had developed their abilities in sensing stress and inactivating their protective processes such as autophagy to fight diseases and live longer.

Autophagy also works to help in the maintenance of homeostasis in your body. During autophagy, your p62 protein helps maintain homeostasis and vibrant health by enabling the damaged cell parts which have accumulated in your body to be turned into new cell formation.

## Ways to Accelerate Autophagy in your Body

There are quite a number of effective ways through which you can expedite the process of autophagy in your body. These are proven methods that you can use to cleanse your cells and reduce your body's inflammation rate to keep your body in pristine condition. However, for the methods to work well, you must trick your body into thinking that it is under immense stress.

## Eating a high-fat and low-carb meal

A diet high in fat and low in carbs is referred to as a keto diet or ketonic diet. Studies show a keto diet helps to accelerate your autophagy processes. Once you adopt a keto diet, your body is forced to shift from burning g glucose to burning fats. The method of burning fats or ketones mimics what happens typically when you are in a fasted state, and this helps to trigger the autophagy process.

You can replace the sugar intake with fat for your life to be transformed through the process of autophagy. The ketonic diet also helps you to lose weight and live a healthy life.

## Go on a protein fast

Another way to accelerate the process of autophagy in your body is by limiting your daily intake of protein. You can start by capping your protein consumption to about 15 to 25 grams per day. Doing this will enable your body to recycle excess proteins. Recycling of excess proteins enables your body to reduce its inflammation rate. Your body will also cleanse its cells even without losing any muscle loss.

During this time, your body will be consuming its protein and toxins through the process of autophagy.

## Practice intermittent fasting

Intermittent fasting is the practice through which you limit the intake of your food for specific periods. Intermittent fasting has been shown to accelerate the process of autophagy in your body significantly. You can accelerate your autophagy processes by skipping your breakfast and then eating generally within eight hours. This kind of fasting will Kickstart and stimulate your body's autophagy processes. Intermittent fasting also enables your body to do a cleanup on all the toxin build-ups in your body.

Moreover, when done effectively, intermittent fasting has been known to cause hormonal imbalance in women. This is because women are naturally susceptible to stressors, such as famine, through starvation or calorie restriction. The hormonal imbalance will then trigger off the process of autophagy. When you keep off any calories, you help your body to attain the fasting state. Your body will then communicate to your cells that it is starving, and the cells will automatically trigger the autophagy process.

Studies also show long fast promotes weight loss and autophagy. When you fast for 24 hours, your body will reverse any loss of stem function. This will enable your body to regenerate itself significantly.

If you are wondering how long you should fast in order to attain autophagy, then most studies agree that a 24-hour period is suitable, although other studies recommend a 16 hour period for your body to trigger autophagy. It has been found that the 16-hour fasting is not as effective as the 24-hour fasting when it comes to autophagy.

## Exercising using high-intensity interval training

You can also stimulate your autophagy by engaging in high-intensity interval training. Such training exposes your body to stress, thus triggering autophagy. You should always remember that autophagy is a natural way through which your body responds to stress. High interval exercises put your body through so much stress that biochemical changes are automatically provoked. Engaging in top impact load exercises will not only make your muscles to be build up but also induce autophagy.

For optimal effect, aim at approximately 20 to 30 minutes of high impact exercises each day. Moreover, experts reckon that you should engage in weight lifting and resistance training exercises for at least 30 minutes each day for your body to effectively Kickstart the process of autophagy. Such exercise usually exposes your body to acute stress. Autophagy loves stress so that the process will be automatically triggered off.

Alternatively, you can engage in other practices involving brisk walking and slow pace walking. This exercise has also been shown to be good at triggering off your autophagy process. Remember to incorporate healthy eating and water intake to your workouts.

## Get enough sleep

Studies show when you get enough sleep, the process of autophagy is highly boosted. Specifically, experts believe that you can activate your autophagy by adopting your body's natural clock or circadian rhythms or sleep-wake cycles. However, you need first to study the four sleep personalities to determine the therapeutic sleep cycle, which works best for you.

You should, therefore, avoid giving up your sleep for your favorite movies or work if you want the process of autophagy to be kick-started in your body.

Studies have revealed that your body works well when you respect its natural clocks or circadian rhythms. Your biological clock usually controls your sleep cycle and patterns. It also influences your autophagy process by controlling it.

When you respect your natural clock, your metabolism process is significantly boosted. While you are asleep, your body makes use of this time to produce and release beneficial hormones. When you deprive yourself of sleep; therefore, you subject it to undue stress, which may have adverse effects on your overall health.

Sleep is very critical in inducing autophagy in your body. Lack of sleep disrupts the process of autophagy or make the process to be prolonged.

## Eat autophagy boosting foods

Certain foods help in accelerating the process of autophagy once you consume them. The following are some of the food that helps to induce your body's cleansing process:

**Coffee-** studies link coffee consumption to the reduction of incidence of metabolic diseases. Coffee is so effective in reducing the metabolic disease because it increases the autophagy process throughout your body. When you consume a single cup of coffee, it leads to a significant increase in autophagy in your liver, heart and muscle cells.

**Ginger-** consumption of ginger can dramatically increase your autophagy. Studies reveal the 6-shogaol components of ginger induces the process of autophagy. The autophagy induced by ginger is so powerful it can destroy a type of lung cancer cells.

**Green tea-**consuming green tea can help induce

your autophagy. Green tea contains some active ingredients called EGCG, which plays a critical role in triggering the process of autophagy in your body. The process is beneficial in fighting inflammation, liver damage, and cancer.

**Coconut oil**- coconut oil contains several ketones. Ketones are the same components that you seek to produce when you engage in fasting. Consuming coconut oil, therefore, will induce autophagy without necessarily starving yourself.

## Using autophagy to get rid of stubborn fats

You can manipulate autophagy to lose stubborn fats in your body. However, you need to understand what triggers the process first. You should also be willing to make the necessary lifestyle for autophagy to work well in helping you to lose the stubborn fats.

When you alter your diet, you help autophagy to fine-tune its processes to effectively get rid of excess fats and make your metabolic processes to be more efficient.

Autophagy can be used to trick your metabolism into working for many hours to burn more fat. The key advantage of this method is that it tends to work at cellular levels and thus produces better and faster results.

For autophagy to work best in increasing your weight loss, you need to incorporate intermittent fasting. This means that you eat a well-planned out diet during a specific window period, and for the rest of the day, you engage in severe fasting for your body to burn the excess fats.

However, before you engage in autophagy fasting, you should seek your doctor's advice on the best diet to follow to achieve better results.

## What SLEEP Got To Do With It

Circadian rhythms and sleep are very important to maximize autophagy. Circadian rhythms refer to the physiological processes of the body that connect with the day and night cycles of your surroundings. The rhythms control the brain, epigenetics, and hormones. Misaligned rhythms are always associated with obesity, diabetes, metabolic syndrome, cancer, depression, and neurodegeneration. This is usually caused by exposure to evening light, which interferes with the circadian clock, and interferes with the quality of sleep.

Deprivation of sleep and poor sleep quality can cause negative health impacts, including Alzheimer's, diabetes, mood disorders, decreased performance, and increased dying risks. Getting quality sleep is the most important means of having a healthy life.

## Autophagy and Sleep

When sleeping, the body undergoes important physiological processes like physical repair, memory consolidation, muscle growth, fat loss, learning new skills, and autophagy. This is the moment when the brain clears out toxic proteins and beta-amyloid, which are associated with autophagy.

Having quality sleep is very crucial in maximizing the benefits of autophagy. The sleep hormone, melatonin, is the one that modulates autophagy. On the other hand, autophagy is also important to get better sleep.

Up to 70% of the pulses of growth hormones

happen during deep sleep. The hormones facilitate regeneration, fat burning, and physical repair. The growth hormones stimulate the liver to initiate autophagy while also supporting the production of glucose.

Can one still gain autophagy with poor sleep? To an extent, gaining autophagy without sleep or with poor sleep quality is possible. However, poor sleep might cause several health conditions. Also, misaligned circadian rhythms also cause stress on the body, thereby preventing one from staying healthy. Nevertheless, restricted feeding within 6 to 8 hours can actually improve one's quality of sleep due to the increased basal level of autophagy.

# CHAPTER:-3

## MAXIMIZING THE EFFECTS OF AUTOPHAGY

Autophagy, though lately rediscovered as a weight management option, has many benefits. It is incredible how a simple change in dietary habits can bring about such a positive difference in one's overall health. It must be noted, though, that autophagy works even better when coupled with exercise. The benefits of one are complemented by the other.

Autophagy occurs when the body 'self-devours' due to a lack of intake of new nutrients. Though it sounds extreme and akin to some sort of cannibalism, it is usually beneficial for cell repair, hormone balancing, improved metabolism, and reduced inflammation. There are a few ways to go about autophagy. These include intermittent fasting, adapting a ketogenic (high fat, low carb) diet, and exercise.

To maximize the results of any given routine, we have to understand the cyclic process of optimization. Let us now look at some of the ways to ensure sustainable results when doing autophagy. This can be summarized in four easy steps, like most processes: identify the problem, engage a plan of action, improve the plan, assess and refine, then repeat.

## Step 1. Identifying The Most Suitable Diet Plan

As with all meaningful practices in life, it is advisable to determine which method of autophagy works best for you and then maintain it. This is the most important step to anchoring your program and ensuring its success. It includes trying out all the available options and finding out which one works best with your body. Establishing a routine takes time, so do not be in a hurry to favor one and discount another. As there are no verified miracles, give yourself time to get used to and adapt the best-suited method for your mind, body, and schedule. It is okay first to try one and then observe the results before you move to the next one.

Ample preparation is advisable when starting any diet plan. The following are suggestions on how to plan, which should make it easy to follow through.

- Discard or give away any snack foods at home or work that may tempt you during your diet

- Create a meal plan, so you know exactly what you're going to eat.

- Tell colleagues, friends, and family that you are likely to see or interact with during this time what you're doing and why it's essential that you have their support

- Arrange to have more time for sleep, as you'll likely be more tired than usual.

- Engage in lighter than usual physical activity on fasting days and any other goal affirming action e.g, listening to a relevant podcast

Consider starting with the easiest and most readily

adaptable one, then move up as your body gets used to the changes. The ketogenic diet would be the most sensible starter diet. The focus of a ketogenic diet is on eating foods that include more fats and fewer carbs. This triggers the same metabolic changes and benefits, sans the fasting. It is more geared towards a person that is not used to skipping meals. In this case, just substitute your regular food intake with items that have higher fat and lower carb content, like eggs, cheese, meat, chicken, avocado, fish, and green leafy vegetables. Steer clear of starches like potatoes, bread, pasta, and sweetened beverages.

Intermittent fasting is the essence of autophagy. This ranges from time-restricted eating, fasting-mimicking diet, alternate-day fasting, to full-day fasting. It is designed to suit and accommodate just about anyone.

Time-restricted eating is basically restricting your eating window to four to five hours a day, and drinking only water or zero-calorie beverages for the rest of the day. The amount of calorie intake in this method is unrestricted within that window. The time frame varies according to the person's preference and the eating plan they choose to follow. This includes eating all the meals and snacks for one day within this period. Some people, however, elect to extend this period up to eight hours and fast for the remaining sixteen. This method is very useful in preventing obesity while maintaining high energy levels throughout the day. It also aids in lowering the risk of diabetes and other metabolic diseases. Persons with diabetes should always seek their doctor's advice before trying this or any other diet program.

A fasting-mimicking diet is a method of triggering autophagy whereby you adhere to a very restricted calorie intake for five days in a week. Ideally, it should be as follows:

**Day 1: 1090 calories, 10% of protein, 56% of fat, 34% of carbs**

**Days 2 up to 5: 725 calories, 9% of protein, 44% of fat, 47% of carbs**

This method tricks your body into believing that you are on an actual fast, thereby enabling you to get the same benefit as if on a real fast while still eating. The benefits derived from this method include sustained weight loss and marked rejuvenation of the immune system. It is considered as a good alternative to complete fasting because it keeps you nourished by continually providing your body with electrolytes and nutrients. You eat tiny portions of easily digestible foods. It is also an easier way to get into prolonged fasting, with less stress to the body. This method, however, takes some time to get used to it. Though some people prefer to do a fasting-mimicking diet at least once a month, it is advisable to do it no less than twice a year.

Alternate day fasting is characterized by fasting one day and eating the next day, and so on. During the fasting days, you consume a total of five hundred calories, of which two hundred are protein. This can be done all in one seating or spaced out throughout the day. You are supposed to drink only water these days. On eating days, you eat your regular portions and may have other drinks in addition to water. It has been found to be a very effective weight-loss tool with reports of up to six percent of the total body weight in a year. It is also a straightforward routine to follow.

Full day fasting is also known as the 5:2 diet. You

eat as usual for five days in the week and have a controlled calorie intake for the other two. On the eating days, you again consume only a total of five hundred calories, of which two hundred are fat. The rest is protein, like fish, nuts, and eggs. It may all be had at once or throughout the day. On eating days you can eat anything you want, at any time, though it is advisable to eat mainly vegetables, fruits, and lean proteins. This is a relatively easy-to-follow diet, especially with people whose daily lives are busy and unpredictable.

While experimenting with all the above methods, consider your safety first. Please keep in mind that any dietary or exercise decisions that will affect your diet and entire wellbeing should first be discussed with your physician. More so if you are pregnant or planning to get pregnant or living with an underlying chronic condition.

## Step 2. Implementing and Maintaining a Routine

Once you have identified which particular type of inducing autophagy works best for you, it is time to come up with a workable routine. The routine you pick should ideally be one that is compatible with your lifestyle and daily schedules. Always keep in mind that your goals should be SMART: Specific, Attainable, Measurable, Realistic, and Time-based. This step is crucial because it ensures that the laid-down plan is correctly followed. It also serves as a reference point for what needs to be done and when. This is until one becomes used to it, and it gets to be like second nature. To properly implement a routine, it is advisable to come up with a list in which you write the daily eating schedule and the required calorie intake of the preferred method. Keep this schedule in a place that is easy to see, for example, the fridge door or the desktop of your computer or phone as opposed to inside a drawer. Also, set a reminder to keep you on track and prevent avoidable lapses in observance of the routine.

For instance, with a current weight of four hundred pounds, a goal to reduce six percent, which translates to twenty-four pounds in one year, is attainable. A workable plan of alternate-day fasting can be put in place and hopefully followed to the letter. With a projected loss of twenty-four pounds in a year, that works out to two pounds per month. Keep a log of your monthly weight and check to see if you are keeping in pace with your projected weight. After the first month, your ideal weight should be 398 pounds, after the second month 396 pounds and so on. By the end of the year, you should weigh 376 pounds. The relatively low figure in proposed weight loss is not overly stressful, and a slight month-to-month delay can easily be corrected. Handled well, one should not feel under pressure. This may be contrasted to wanting to lose fifty pounds within the year, which would translate to losing slightly over four pounds a month. Failure to achieve this may make one feel distressed, frustrated, and likely to give up. The above is only an example and not endorsed by any physician whatsoever.

They say that anything worth achieving takes time, and in a way, this is also a chance to cultivate patience too.

## Step 3. Engaging in Complementary Exercise

Exercise is a trigger for autophagy in its own right. Regular exercise is an unintentional way in which people help their bodies to cleanse themselves. When we exercise, tiny tears form in our muscles, and the body rushes to heal them, resulting in stronger and more tear-resistant muscles. In mice, autophagy during exercise was noted to be at its peak between thirty to eighty minutes on a treadmill. It is not yet clear how this translates to humans, but it is a clear indication of the relationship between autophagy and exercise. Exercise has also been shown to decrease insulin levels and increase glucagon levels, which then induces autophagy. Combining exercise and a diet/fasting plan is a sure way to see a marked and sustained improvement in overall health. Remember, as you shed the pounds, you will need to firm up your body. Therefore it is advisable to find an exercise routine that will match up with your chosen diet. Treadmill exercise has been noted to be very effective as a trigger for autophagy, and it is easy enough to do, on any diet. Pair lighter exercises with fasting days and moderate to high-intensity exercise with eating days.

For instance, on fasting days, do a thirty-minute treadmill exercise or workout divided into ten minutes each, with an emphasis on cardio. On the other hand, on eating days, do your regular work out of perhaps one hour or more, including cardio, resistance, and strength training. Be careful not to over-exercise. Too much exercise leads to overtraining syndrome, which is detrimental to your health. It has adverse effects such as hormonal imbalance, reduced immunity, fatigue, difficulty sleeping, increased stress and restlessness, among others.

## Step 4. Reviewing and Adjusting the Routine

After having used your routine of choice for a specific period, say two months, take a look back and assess how it is working for you. Be very honest with yourself in regards to the intended goal as recorded in your schedule, and the achievement realized during the assessment.

If any shortcomings are noticed, find a way to adjust the routine or your expectations and keep at it. Sometimes a whole new system, which means an overhaul and change from the current method to another, may be necessary. The critical thing to keep in mind is that the ultimate goal is your wellbeing and the role that renewed and repaired cells in your body play towards that. This should be enough of a motivation to keep you going and trying out new ways until you find one that works best for you without unduly stressing you. Be careful, also, not to overdo any of the above techniques, as there are possible downsides too. The most prevalent of these is malnutrition due to abstaining for food for too long, which leads to starvation. This, in turn, causes the body's systems to slow down and hence reduced muscle mass and inefficient metabolism. Moderation is key to going about autophagy, as well as everything else in life. Try not to do too little, but also learn to cut back and recalibrate when it turns out that you are doing too much.

As we said earlier, optimization is a process. As such, once you have reviewed your routine and identified the problem areas in the method or combination of techniques that you are using, make the necessary adjustments and go back to step 1 or 2, as needed. Habitually check on your progress and modify it continually. Achieving perfection is desirable, though not always attainable. The very act of continual improvement gets us closer to the ultimate goal.

Finally, it is worth noting too that no single method will work for everyone. As such, what works for your friend, colleague, or family member will not necessarily work for you. Do not let that discourage you. Keep trying, find your rhythm, and settle into a routine that you are comfortable with, without allowing external pressures to affect your morale or drive. You are in charge of your own decisions and destiny. Make it work and make it count!

## Keeping Up with the Latest Research

Autophagy, in the form of fasting, has been touted and practiced in one way or the other by most religions for millennia. These include Judaism, Christianity, Buddhism, Hinduism, and Baha'i. Only now has science caught up with and put emphasis on the benefits likely to be derived from autophagy, most notably through different forms of fasting and exercise. A lot of research still needs to be done on autophagy and how it impacts our health. So far, research shows that autophagy is good for our health. The continual cell regeneration and renewal has been documented to be advantageous in various fields. These include cancer prevention and management, reduced risk of neurodegenerative diseases, improved muscle performance, better digestive health, and skin health, fighting infectious diseases, supporting a healthy weight, and even some anti-aging benefits. Everyone should try autophagy. Nutrition and health experts agree that there is yet much to be learned about autophagy, its benefits, and implementation on a large scale. Scientists are even working on pills to imitate the effects of a ketogenic diet though it is currently used to treat epilepsy.

Given the above, it is advisable to keep current with advances in the up-and-coming field of autophagy. Hopefully, in the near future, it will be possible to implement it on a large scale, starting with the younger generation. This will encourage them to grow up with and carry forth healthy living practices to the next generation and posterity.

# CHAPTER:-4

## INTERMITTENT FASTING AND AUTOPHAGY

Intermittent fasting involves going without food for a while days. This period is, however, undefined. There are many documented health benefits of intermittent fasting that make it such a common practice for those who are keen at preventing lifestyle diseases such as heart disease, diabetes, and cancer. Intermittent fasting is also helpful in speeding the process through which your body loses fat. Moreover, intermittent fasting plays a key to slowing or reversing your aging process.

This kind of fasting also reduces inflammation and oxidative stress leading to an increase in the number and quality of mitochondria. This increases an internal process called autophagy. Autophagy is the process

47

through which the cellular system cleans itself to get rid of harmful oxidants.

## How Intermittent Fasting Works

There are quite a number of physiological processes involved in intermittent fasting to work effectively. Of importance is that the many health benefits resulting from this type of fasting come as a result of the reduction of insulin in your body.

The critical function of insulin in your body is to facilitate the storage of energy and the growth of the organism. An increase in insulin level leads to an increase in the fats stored in the fatty cells. Besides, the increase in insulin leads to more cells taking up glucose from your blood. The rise of fat in your cells is often blamed for many health problems.

Moreover, an increase in insulin results in the fatty lipids depositing in the fat cells. You need, therefore, to pay a lot of attention to your diet, exercise, and fasting to lose the excess fat in the cells by getting the lipids out of fat cells to be burned.

## How Intermittent Fasting Lowers Insulin

## Level to Help Autophagy

One of the critical effects of intermittent fasting is the lowering of the insulin level in your body. The low insulin level, on the other hand, increases lipolysis. The success of this process, however, depends on several factors. Top among this is the duration you need to fast for your insulin levels to fall.

Moreover, eating usually causes insulin levels in your body to rise. The amount of the rise depends on such factors as the type of food you consume, the amount of that food, and how sensitive your body is to the insulin.

Eating food with a high amount of carbohydrates usually lowers your insulin sensitivity dramatically. When your insulin sensitivity is reduced, the production of insulin in your body rises. Therefore, low insulin sensitivity results in an automatic rise in insulin levels in your body.

Besides, after eating, your insulin levels shoot up and stay high for several hours. This is what is referred to as the fed state. When fasting, you consume little or no amounts of food, therefore, lowering your insulin levels.

## What Time Does Intermittent Fasting Work Best for Autophagy

The best duration for intermittent fasting to work well is between 18 to 24 hours of fasting. Studies show when you fast for this period, you will experience the most considerable drop in your insulin level, and your lipolysis process is drastically increased.

However, most people are not comfortable fasting for so long. At some point, you may be overwhelmed with hunger even when you desperately want to lose weight. The realistic duration, therefore, which can work well for you, is fasting for about 16 hours. A 16 hour fast means you skip only one meal. You may choose to skip breakfast, making your fasting quite easy and comfortable.

But, if you can extend your fast further to the afternoon, then you stand to gain even more benefits. You achieve more significant results with a 24 hour fast.

You should take into consideration that the duration of the fast is key to achieving autophagy. It is not about attaining low insulin levels only, but how long can you sustain the low levels of insulin in your body. You should, therefore, aim at fasting for more extended periods, although you may experience a lot of challenges in terms of convenience in going about your normal life while on the fast.

## Autophagy: The Connection between Intermittent Fasting and Autophagy

Autophagy is the natural process through which your body's system cleans itself. Your body cells create membranes that locate and get rid of dead, diseased, or worn-out cells and use the resultant molecules for energy or to recreate new cell parts. It is a natural way through which our bodies recycle the waste. Autophagy is beneficial to you because the process gets rid of faulty parts and, most importantly, stops cancerous growths. It also prevents or lowers metabolic dysfunctions, such as diabetes and obesity.

Autophagy also plays a critical role in controlling inflammation and immunity of your body. A study of rats that were incapable of autophagy showed that they were much fatter, sleepier, and had high levels of cholesterol with impaired brain functions. Autophagy is also beneficial in lowering your aging process, making you looked younger than your real age. One of the ways to achieve autophagy is through intermittent fasting. So how is this possible? You ask yourself.

Well, when you restrict your calorie intake for an extended period, you gain a lot of health benefits. Such benefits include weight loss, longer life, and changes to risk factors for heart disease and diabetes.

There are a lot of studies done to establish the link between fasting and longevity in life. In a study done on lab mice, it was found that fasting mice for periods increase the tendency for them to live longer than their other peers who eat normally.

Researchers sought an explanation for this, and they concluded that when you restrict your calorie intake, your genes that tell cells to preserve resources are turned on. In turn, the cells go into a preservation mode or a famine mode. This mode makes the cells to be much more resistant to diseases or cellular stress. The cells also initiate autophagy, where the body cleans itself by getting rid of old, unwanted, and diseased cellular material. It also recycles any damaged parts.

In yet another study done on lab mice, the mice were fasted by 24 hours to establish the effect of fasting on their autophagy. The study showed that the mice increased their number of autophagosomes substantially after the fast. This was a reliable indicator that fasting plays a significant role in autophagy. However, it is a challenge measuring autophagy outside the lab environment because the metabolism process in humans' is much slower than the one done on mice, but still many experts believe that the autophagy process is triggered off in humans after 18 to 20 hours of fasting, with the maximal benefit is expected to be realized once you reach a 48-72-hour mark.

It is advisable, therefore, to consider a more extended period of fast to fully activate autophagy that is beneficial in the cleaning of your body cells. However, you should always seek your doctor's advice before you adopt any fasting regime, especially if you have any health risk factors.

Once you stimulate autophagy, several things take place in your body. First, old, unwanted cellular materials and protein are cleared out. Besides, autophagy will also stimulate the production of growth hormones in your body. The growth hormone plays a critical role in the regeneration of fresh cellular materials. It also initiates the cell renewal in your body. Autophagy also improves your immune system by destroying any traces of bacteria or virus, especially if your body had a recent infection.

Moreover, fasting to achieve autophagy has helped researchers to understand degenerative diseases such as Alzheimer's, cancer, and Parkinson's. Failure for autophagy to take place regularly results in your body accumulating different kinds of cellular material, which show up in large quantities in Alzheimer's, cancer, and Parkinson's persons.

Researchers hold the belief that if you go through autophagy for long periods, the development of these diseases, especially cancer, will be stopped. This is possible with the clearance of excess protein in your brain through autophagy.

## How to Achieve Autophagy Through Fasting

There are several myths doing rounds on how you

can effectively make autophagy. Some of these myths are not only unproven but also based on blatant lies. There is, however, one sure way through which you can make autophagy. And that is through fasting.

There are two ways through which your body benefits from fasting to achieve autophagy. These are the pathways that make your body to deplete their nutrients.

The first one is the mTOR, also known as the mammalian target of rapamycin. When you eat a lot of carbs, the production of insulin in your body is triggered. Insulin, on the other hand, triggers protein synthesis through a kinase. This process is what is commonly referred to as mammalian TOR or mTOR. An increase in mammalian TOR leads to the suppression of autophagy. Therefore, fasting is key to lowering the mammalian TOR to increase autophagy. This theory has been backed up by mice trials and in-vitro human trials. The tests gave credence to the conclusion that fasting actually stimulates autophagy in human beings.

The second one is called AMPK or AMP-activated

kinase. This is the process through which your body is aided to maintain energy homeostasis. Your body also activates the fuel back up a mechanism through this process.

mTOR and AMK are highly familiar with and sensitive to the presence of nutrients in your body. They also play an important role in making your body either to activate a growth response or to go into autophagy. In fact, during the fed state, the rate of autophagy in your body is quite low. However, during the fasting period, autophagy increases significantly as your insulin levels drop. Some people have experienced an increase in autophagy levels of up to 5-fold during their fasting period.

Researchers also believe that the several anti-aging effects of calorie restriction and intermittent fasting come as a result of the increase in autophagy. A high rate of autophagy is common to young organisms. As you age, the rate of autophagy decreases significantly, allowing for the accumulation of cellular damage. But when you fast intermittently, the rate of autophagy is reset to the level of a young person.

Besides, autophagy also works in tandem with two critical hormones. These are insulin and glucagon. If you are suffering from hypoglycemia or diabetes, you may experience some challenges regulating your insulin levels. You may also be overly sensitive to insulin in your body. Whenever insulin rises in your body, the levels of glucagon drops significantly and vice versa. When you fast, you tend to lower the insulin levels in your body and increase the levels of glucagon. This will automatically stimulate autophagy.

You should also note the importance of exercise to fasting and autophagy. Physical exercises are known to improve the sensitivity of your insulin. When you fast and practice a healthy exercise routine, the levels of your insulin will tend to drop significantly, and the lipolysis process is triggered off after as compared to someone who fails to incorporated exercise into their fasting routine.

Another factor to note is the role of a low carbohydrate diet in fasting and autophagy. When you consume low carbs diets and then engage in intermittent fasting, you will experience a faster drop in your insulin levels. This promotes a faster lipolysis process and autophagy.

It is also important to note that autophagy is often suppressed by the presence of insulin resistance in your body and hyperinsulinemia. Exercise and intermittent fasting much help to overcome this challenge by making your body to be highly sensitive to insulin leading to an increase in autophagy.

However, intermittent fasting is not easy to achieve. It needs a lot of commitments and discipline on your part to induce autophagy through fasting. You need to make low levels of liver glycogen, which usually takes place after 14-16 hours of fasting for your body to Kickstart the process of autophagy. This, however, is more likely to happen after 24 hours of serious fasting.

However, the level of fasting for you to activate autophagy varies with individuals. Some tend to experience some side effects such as moodiness, feelings of low energy, and insomnia during the time of fasting. It is essential, therefore, to always seek your health care provider's advice before you embark on intermittent fasting.

# Types of Intermittent Fasting to Help Autophagy

Intermittent fasting has become quite popular across the globe. The proponents of this kind of fasting claim it leads to rapid weight loss, improves your metabolic health, and even extends your lifespan. New studies have given credence to these claims, with several proving that those who practice intermittent fasting experience higher rates of autophagy.

As a result of this popularity, several types of intermittent fasting schedules have been developed. Although all are effective, you should choose one which suits your individual needs without causing any side effects. Here are some of the common ways to do intermittent fasting:

## 16/8 Method of Intermittent Fasting

Choosing this method, means you are ready to fast for up to 16 hours each day. You fast for 14 hours to a maximum of 16 hours each day as you restrict your eating window to only 8-10 hours daily.

Within this eating window, you can choose to schedule 2 to 3 meals depending on your needs.

59

This method, which is also known as the Leangains protocol, is quite popular with health enthusiasts who are keen at increasing their autophagy. It is as simple as skipping after-dinner snacks as well as skipping your breakfast.

A good example would be you eat your dinner at 8 pm and avoid eating anything until midday the following day. You would have succeeded in fasting for 16 hours between your meals.

However, women are advised to fast for 14-15 hours only. This is because their autophagy process seems to be active with shorter fasts.

You are allowed to drink non-caloric beverages such as water, coffee, or tea during your fasting period. This will significantly help in reducing your thirst and hunger pangs. It is also advisable to eat healthy foods during your window period. You should, therefore, avoid any junk food and unhealthy fats. Instead, go for healthy servings such as vegetables and whole grains with a lot of water.

## The 5:2 Intermittent Fasting

This type of fasting involves eating for five days while fasting for two days of the week. During your fasting period, you are required to restrict your calorie consumption to between 500 and 600 calories. The 5:2 diet is also called a Fast diet and needs women to eat 500 calories, and while men consume 600 calories during their two-day fasting period each week.

An excellent example of this fasting routine is when you choose to eat normally on all the days of the week except on Tuesdays and Fridays. On these two days, you decide to eat smaller meals of 250 calories per meal for men and 300 calories per meal for the women. Although the effectiveness of this kind of diet has been subjected to many debates, the two-day fasting comes with a lot of health benefits to those who practice it.

## Eat Stop Eat Intermittent Fasting

This kind of diet expects you to do a 24 hour fast, once or two times each week. The popularity of this method has been rising over the last few years. You can choose to achieve a 24 hour fast by fasting after dinner on Mondays until dinner on the following day. You may also want to fast from one breakfast to another.

For example, you finish your breakfast on Monday morning and avoid any food until the breakfast of the following day.

However, you are allowed to take water and other non-caloric beverages during your fasting period. It is also important to eat normally during your eating periods. You should eat the same quantity of the food as you usually consume when you are not fasting.

However, many people find a full 24 hour fast to be quite challenging. You can, therefore, choose to start with a shorter period of 14 to 16 hours before you move upwards to fasting for a full 24 hours. You also need a lot of discipline and commitment to successfully carry out this kind of fasting.

## Alternate Day Intermittent Fasting

In this kind of diet, you are expected to alternate your fasting periods such that you fast after every other day. This fasting has several different versions. Some restrict your calorie intake to 500 during your fasting days. You also need to be well prepared for this fast because you are likely to go to bed hungry several times each week. This can be quite unpleasant and unsustainable over the long run.

## The Intermittent Warrior Diets

The warrior diet involves fasting during the day and eating a huge meal during the night. Alternatively, you can choose to eat some small amounts of raw fruits and vegetables during the day and eating a big meal at night. It merely means you fast during day time, and you feast at night. You should also give yourself a 4-hour window period between day time and night time meals. This kind of diet was one of the intermittent pioneer diets popular with many people.

This diet also encourages the consumption of food choices, similar to a paleo diet. Paleo diets are whole, unprocessed foods with the same similarity to what they look like in nature.

## Spontaneous Dieting

This kind of diet involves the skipping of meals whenever it is convenient for you. There is no structured fasting plan that you follow, you just avoid food whenever it is suitable for you to do so.

You can skip food occasionally, especially when you

are not feeling hungry or whenever you are too busy to cook or eat. It is a fallacy that you must eat at specific times of the day in order not to starve. Your body is well equipped to endure long periods of famine, and skipping one or two meals occasionally can present no health risks.

You can quickly and comfortably skip breakfast whenever you are not hungry and choose to eat one meal either during lunch hour or dinner time. If you skip 1 or 2 meals whenever it is convenient for you, you are merely engaging in intermittent fasting.

Finally, intermittent fasting is not for the lose hearted. However, it is something you need to do to increase your autophagy. This kind of fasting is quite beneficial for both men and women. However, you should seek advice from your health care providers before engaging in intermittent fasting, especially if you have some underlying health conditions. If you finally decide to go intermittent fasting way, then keep in mind that you need to incorporate a good work out regime and eat healthy to maximize its benefits and increase your autophagy.

If You like this book, I would be very grateful if You leave a short review on Amazon.

# CHAPTER:-5

## CHOOSING THE RIGHT FASTING TYPE

When you think of losing weight, then you have to prepare your mind and try to add more energy, look no further than fasting. When you lower your risks for ailments and enhance your memory, you will be able to have the fun of health benefits by having a change when you feed. There have been fasting diets that have been there for many decades, and nowadays, the trending fasting components are the paleo and keto. You will be able to get a fasting regimen that suits you, depending on how you feed and plan your health goals. Fasting fits into any diet, but you can enhance more structure because you have alternatives.

Never think fasting is all about religious

determinations. There is a new phenomenon that is helping in weight loss known as the Intermittent Fasting (IF), and it is becoming popular in health and appropriateness trends. When using IF, you have to alternate amid the times you are eating and fasting. This can be referred to as patterns or cycles of fasting. You can use various types of ways to IF, but they will all come down to individual variance. You have to know what will work out the best for you when you have any intentions of trying the IF. For the first time, there may be trial and error. Many people have it easy to fast for 16 hours and curb meals to just 8 hours of the day. Some people, at the same time, will have hard times prefer to shorten their fasting window.

## Are You Doing Well with Intermittent Fasting?

There has been a study showing the positive impacts of IF like weight loss, low blood pressure, and enhanced metabolic health, but still, there is a need for investigations about the long-term outcomes of IF. You can also look at the aspect of sustainability. When restricting or not feeding on calories for some time, it is not the same for everyone. Study as also shown that those using intermittent fasting rarely stick to it, unlike those using traditional diets to weight loss.

Even still, IF it has been the best effective form when it comes to weight loss. There are also other methods like feeding on a well-balanced diet alongside exercises. There is also another study that showed IF is not the best when it comes to weight loss or enhancing blood sugars. When you want to lose weight, then you should know that it is not a one size fit all tactic. IF is sustainable to specific groups of people, but others find this process not right for them. For you to try IF, then, you have to know how will you fix this feeding in your life, and this is when it comes to issues like social functions and trying to be active. There are some known IF methods, as explained below.

## 1. The Twice a Week Technique – 5:2

This kind of tactic to IF will assist you in covering your calories at 500 for two days in a week. The remaining five days of the week, you will have to stick to a healthy diet as always. When on fasting occasions, then this tactic has an inclusion of 200-calorie meals and a 300-calorie meal. You must concentrate on foods with high fiber and protein to help you fill up and keep calories low as you are fasting. You are free to take any two fasting days as long as there is a day you are not fasting between them. And remember always to eat the same amount of food you feed on regular non-fasting days.

## 2. Alternate Fasting Days

This kind of variation has involved a modified fasting every single day. For example, you can control your calories on the days you are fasting to 500 or 25% of your regular consumption. Days when you are not fasting, you have to go back to your daily and healthy feeding habits. You can also encounter some strict variations that entail the consumption of 0 calories on substitute days as a replacement of 500. There is another study that shows people who follow this form of IF in a retro of six months has suggestively raised cholesterol levels after six months off the diet.

## 3. Restricted Time of Eating

When using this method, you to set fasting and eating windows. For instance, you can fast for 16 hours of your day, and you can feed for only eight hours of the day. Most of the time, people fast when they are sleeping, and this is a popular method. This can be

69

operative because you will extend overnight fasting when you skip breakfast, and you are not eating until you get to lunchtime. There are popular ways like:

- 16/8 process: this is when you eat only between 11 a.m. and 7 p.m. or amid noon and 8 p.m.

- 14/10 method: this is when you only feed between 10 a.m. and 8 p.m.

This method you can try and repeat it as many times, or you can do it once or twice a week. This depends on your personal preference. When you get the right eating and fasting windows for this process, it can take you some days to find out, and this can work out when you are active, or you start your day hungry for breakfast. This kind of fasting is safe for a lot of people who have an interest in trying IF for the first time.

## 4. 24 Hours Fasting

This is a method that you have to fast fully for 24 hours. This will be done most of the time, once or twice a week. You can decide to fast from breakfast to breakfast or lunch at lunch. This kind of version of IF has some side effects that can be risky, like being tired, aches, irritation, hunger, and low energy. When you are following this process, then you have to return to a normal and healthy diet on the days you are not fasting.

## Intermittent Fasting Isn't a Magic Pill

Whether you are using IF, keto, low carbohydrates, high protein, among others, they will all come down to the eminence of your calories and the amount you are incontrollable. What you have to know about IF is that; however, the jury is still out, and long-term effects are being investigated, you will be required to have a healthy and well-balanced diet when you are using IF. You are not able to lose or reduce weight when feeding on junk foods and excess calories on the days you are not fasting.

## Side Effects and the Risks

This kind of fasting may not be safe for some people, such as pregnant women, children, or someone with some chronic illness. In cases that you have some feeding disorder, you are advised not to try any fasting diet. IF can increase the likelihood of binge feeding on other people due to limitations. If you are interested in trying the IF fasting, then you should be aware of some small side effects that will come along. IF can be partnered with touchiness, low or lack of energy, persistent hunger, sensitivity in temperature, and poor working and activity presentation.

## Where to Begin?

You should put into consideration some simple form of IF when you are beginning. If you want to start IF, then its recommended to start with a moderate approach and restrict eating time. You should start by cutting out your nighttime feeding and snacking, and then you will go ahead to limit your daily food like eating from 8 a.m. to 6 p.m. when progressing and checking how you are feeling, you can decide to upsurge your fasting period. You should speak by a doctor or dietician before you begin using IF fasting. You have to take caution and go slow with it.

Intermittent fasting can be like the current buzzworthy health fad that will assist when it comes to losing weight, but professionals say it is not hype. A lot of professionals have recommended that the diet can help in boosting longevity and maintaining blood sugar levels and healthy weight. You can think that too fast is all about skipping meals and upping your intake of water. There are a lot of processes of IF fasting that can be used in any lifestyle. You can try to break down the kind of forms that can work or won't work.

## 1:1 Process the Least Sustainable Fasting Process

This is the least successful variation of fasting, which is known as the 1:1 method or alternative fasting. This kind of fasting is where you have regular feeding for 24 hours and then fast on the next. This can be applied once or twice a week. This process has been considered to be popular to kick start loss of weight; this can be least sustainable compared to all the fasting methods and in the long run, has been associated with eating a lot of food when you are not fasting.

## 16:8 Process of Fasting

This kind of approach will require you to eat for eight hours a day and then go ahead and fats for 16 hours a day. This is one of the most accessible forms of IF that you can maintain because you can feed daily, and there are a lot of meals that you can eat within eight hours. You can adjust the period to meet your lifestyle wants and characters.

Warrior nourishment will allow you to eat some fruits and vegetables when you are fasting. When you are on a warrior diet, you may tend to eat fruits, vegetables, and take liquids that have zero calories for 20 hours daily. When you are maintaining this kind of diet, you should be allowed to carry large amounts of food in the evening. This kind of diet will require you to have more focus on the quality of your diet, and this won't be sustainable to you most of the time.

Generally, IF is preferred to be the best for your gut. Intermittent fasting has been capable of increasing bacterial variety and has inclined the balance of valuable gut bacteria that can assist your body against obesity and increase of weight. Some people always think that intermittent fasting has several verdicts. Current research has shown that IF has diverse findings and won't appear to give compelling metabolic or weight loss advantages to the traditional calorie restraint.

IF it is complicated to maintain for an extended period, even though the method that you will take this kind of process will be hard to keep up with for a long time, this can be so to someone who likes to eat every time. When you have decided you will be using intermittent fasting, then you are supposed to consult with a dietitian. Fasting is not for everyone like pregnant women are not advised to practice this process. Some people also take their medication with food and such cases you will be required to adjust your feeding window to curb in your wants.

Don't feel discouraged, and try to move to a different kind of fasting procedure. The best thing you can do is to get your preferred method and stick to it, and you should not feel afraid to move to another protocol in cases where you find an original choice that you think won't match your lifestyle. The benefits are worth your efforts, and when you try and fail, then be sure there will result soon.

## Health Benefits of Intermittent Fasting

When you are talking about weight loss, then you have to put some thoughts about why IF can work.

When you first fast, there will be a reduction in the net calorie intake; thus, you will lose weight. Some of the benefits of intermittent fasting include:

## Weight loss

Most people consider intermittent fasting with the aim of losing weight. In an article published by the *Journal of the Academy of Nutrition and Dietetics* in 2015, there are high chances that intermittent fasting contributes to weight loss. The study looked at data involving 13 studies and revealed that weight loss witnessed from the program ranged from 1.3% to 8% for a 2-weeks and 8-weeks trial.

It is clear that the amount of weight loss through intermittent fasting does not seem to be more than what one would expect in a calorie-restricted diet. Also, weight loss is dependent on the total calories one takes every day.

## Reduced blood pressure

Intermittent fasting can help you lower your blood pressure. In a Nutrition and Healthy Aging study published in 2018, it was found that 16:8 fasting reduced the systolic blood pressure in 23 participants.

Having healthy blood pressure is keyto avoiding diseases like stroke, heart disease, and kidney disease.

## Reduced inflammation

Studies involving animals have shown that both calorie restriction and intermittent fasting can help reduce the levels of inflammation. A study published by Nutrition Research involving 50 participants who fasted for Ramadan found that there were lower pro-inflammatory markers as well as low body weight, body fat, and blood pressure.

## Lower cholesterol

In a 3-weeks long study published by the journal, Obesity, alternate-day fasting may help in lowering cholesterol levels and LDL cholesterol when done with endurance exercise. LDL cholesterol is known to be bad cholesterol which can increase the risk of stroke and other heart-related diseases. The Centers for Diseases Control and Prevention also noted that intermittent fasting can reduce the presence of triglycerides, fats that are found in the blood that can cause heart attack, heart diseases, and stroke.

## Boosts brain function

What is good for the body is also healthy for the brain. When you do intermittent fasting, you will be able to improve your metabolic features, including reduced inflammation, reduced oxidative stress, and insulin resistance. Different studies in rats have shown that fasting increases the growth of nerve cells that benefits the brain. It also showed that intermittent fasting increased the levels of the brain hormone, brain-derived neurotrophic factor (BDNF), whose deficiency is implicated in depressive symptoms.

## Protection against cancer

Studies have shown that intermittent fasting, particularly alternate-day fasting, can reduce the risk of cancer through the decrease in the development of lymphoma, slowing down the spread of cancer cells. A review study published by the *American Journal of Clinical Nutrition* also found that cancer benefits were observed in all animal studies conducted, which confirmed the benefits for humans.

## People Who Should Not Try Intermittent Fasting

It is not advisable for everyone to try IF. This is

because you can be in periods where you are not supposed to eat, yet you have some illness that can lead to a dangerous path to decline. The type of people who are not supposed to practice this method is pregnant women, those going medication on diabetes, someone on drugs, or someone with eating disorders.

You should be able to note that IF has side effects. You maybe feel cranky or hanger when you are fasting, and this may be due to low blood sugar levels that can interfere with your moods. You are advised to be on a healthy diet when you are not fasting. It can be tiring to make up for a calorie deficit if you have fasted for two days, but in the current society, you can access calorie-dense items that can be able to do it as suggested by professionals. You can maintain nutrient-packed choices like fruits, lean meats, vegetables, grains. For the first couple of weeks, you will have to deal with lower energy, inflating, and desires until when your body adapts to the process.

A lot of people will want to eat what the dietitian has told them. But with time, most people visit them to inquire about what not to eat. IF diet is the solution to weight loss, excellent metabolic health, and health and longer life. Before you start to give up on foods for some days to increase the process of weight loss, then you have to put this into consideration: the medical and nutritionist experts that have to advise you about fasting and weight loss. They will tell you about focusing on enhancing a balanced diet, then you will have to get the experience of starvation, and with so much care, you are allowed to try the practice.

Intermittent fasting has been considered to be a worldwide known health and fitness trend. A lot of people have opted to use it to reduce or lose weight; thus, this improves their health and simplifies their routines. IF has been suggested by a study that it has some powerful effects on your body and brain; therefore, this can make you have a longer life.

# CHAPTER:-6

## THINGS TO KEEP IN MIND DURING FASTING

Fasting or intermittent fasting as it popularly is known is the new trend in town. It merely involves choosing what time to eat while ensuring you remain fast for the other periods. It doesn't mean that you fail to eat, or you keep count of your calorie intake or even restrict what you eat. It is a newly found freedom of choosing what you eat and at what time you eat it. It is a simple, inexpensive way to help you stay healthy and look younger.

Interment fasting has been proven to have a lot of health benefits, especially to those who have diabetes or have been considered pre-diabetes by their doctors. To them, it helps lose weight as well as reduce insulin resistance in their bodies, thus making the medication

81

they are receiving more effective. This way, the body can regulate their glucose levels, protecting them from the harmful effects of hyperglycemia. Other health benefits include but are not limited to a reduction in blood pressure, detoxification, and slowing down the aging process.

You have probably been considering intermittent fasting as your dietary choice for some time now. But the challenge is you do not know where to start, what to do, and how to tell whether your fasting is being successful or not. You have asked your friends or staring on the internet about it, but you still cannot find a suitable answer for yourself. Nothing seems to give you clear cut instructions on what to do, what to avoid, and when to know whether you have surpassed your limits. Worry no more, for in this chapter, we will discuss tips for a successful fast and what you should consider before you begin fasting.

## Tips for Successful Fasting

We have already discovered the potential benefits of fasting and are ready to kick start our journey. What we do not know is that fasting done wrong can expose you to health risks, including hypoglycemia, fatigue, weakness, and even coma most likely for those who have diabetes. The different types of fasting have been discussed and before you chose the most appropriate one for you, here are a few tips to ensure your fasting is successful;-

## 1. Ensure you adequately prepare your body

Imagine today you are told that you are to run the world marathon of just 3kms. At first, you would be super excited, but then the excitement dwindles once you realize the amount of work that is ahead of you before you can consider yourself ready to run. You would need to need to build your stamina and endurance by training for long hours and watching what you eat. It's the same context when you are considering beginning fasting. In simple terms, fasting is like running the marathon. You need to prepare your body for the tough times ahead. Slowly cut down the amount of food that you consume per day. This way, your body starts adapting to using lesser calories for survival gradually. Then cut down on all sugars and finally processed foods that you consume daily. This way, you begin to cleanse your body of all the waste food it has been consuming over time in a bid to detoxify your body. Instead, I now concentrate on consuming raw fruits and vegetables and whole grains. These foods are rich in enzymes and nutrients that you require to heal and function optimally. Also, by providing the body with plenty of proteins before the fast, it ensures your body is ready to focus on improving itself.

It is essential to understand that though some people require time to get into fasting, some can jump right into it without detrimental health effects.

## 2. Stay hydrated

Your body derives 20 to 30 percent of its total water from the food you consume. It, therefore, means that during fasting, your body is deficient in water. Thus, researchers recommend that you take up to 8 ounces of water per day during fasting. This way, you stay hydrated and provide adequate water for your cells to function optimally. Water is also crucial in helping get rid of toxins from the body. Dehydration can cause detrimental effects on your body, including fatigue, headaches, and dry mouth. But how do you know that you are taking adequate water? The color of your urine gives a lot of information about the state of your health, hydration status being one of them. Your urine should be clear though some vitamins like Vitamin D may cause the urine to be yellow despite taking plenty of water.

### 3. Keep your fasting periods short

Popular fasting regimens have already been discussed. You could choose to fast for 12hours a day or 16 hours or the whole 24hours. Or you could choose to fast two days in a week or alternate days of the week. Another fasting technique is where you decide to skip meals within a day. Either way, you will be doing intermittent fasting, and you will experience similar benefits so long as you follow the rules for each technique. Most of the fasting regimens recommend fasting between 6 to 48 hours though some people choose to go for as long as 72 hours. Longer fasting hours are associated with an increased risk of experiencing side effects, which include dehydration, mood swings, irritability, fainting, and inability to concentrate. To protect yourself from this, choose the regimen that is most suitable for you. One that you will be able to continue with work as usual without experiencing the unwanted side effects or being uncomfortable. It is advisable that if you choose to fast for more than 72 hours, you seek medical advice, especially if you already have a medical condition.

## 4. Distract yourself

In the first few days after you begin your fasting, your energy levels will be low, and all you will think about is food. You will want to damn the whole process and eat a burger or some other tempting food. You will not want to participate in any activity as a result of your plunged moods and energy levels. But as the days continue, your body will get used to it, and your energy levels will return to normal. You will be the vibrant individual you were as before, and food will be the last thing on your mind. However, the transition will not smooth. You will so much be tempted to eat mostly when you see your friends going to get food. You will want to join them. It is very normal. You will require a lot of discipline during this period. You will need to keep yourself busy during these periods. Clear out the stack of files on your desk, clean out your

86

house, or take a walk. When you see your friends going for lunch, no matter how tempting it is, say no and go ahead to find something else to do to keep your mind off food. Whatever it is you do, ensure you keep yourself busy and distracted.

## 5. Avoid binge eating

It is the period after your fast, and it is time for you to eat again. It is time you have been eagerly waiting for the past 6 to 72 hours. All your body is doing is asking for food. It wants food, and it wants it badly. You cannot wait to get those fries and burgers that your body is yearning. But wait a minute. Is this the right way to break a fast? And how exactly should I break a fast? Well, take small light meals to break your fast. Take a small light meal immediately, and then if you feel hungry, you could eat another one. Avoid binge eating, which is taking dense unhealthy foods all at once. They not only leave you feeling guilty but leave you bloated and tired. They also make your body feel overwhelmed after a period of break, leaving you feeling slow and sleepy. One thing you will notice after your period of fasting, it that you require lesser food than before to get satisfied despite your brain telling

87

you to eat more. It is because fasting causes your stomach to grow smaller. However, your brain does not adapt as fast, and it will be the one telling you to eat more. That is why you must listen to your body and stop eating when it says so.

## 6. Eat more proteins

Most people start fasting as a way of losing weight. It works by creating an energy deficit in your body by providing minimal calories. This way, the body due to lack of glucose, which is generally utilized as a source of energy, the body starts breaking down fats stored in the body for energy. This way, the excess fats around the tummy and hips are broken down, giving you a slimmer sexier look. What most do not understand is that the body breaks down protein, in this case, muscle, together with the fats. It could lead to muscle loss and actual starvation. Therefore, you must take plenty of proteins during your fasting breaks to try and prevent breaking down of muscle during your fasting hours. In addition to preventing muscle loss, proteins also have additional benefits, including regulating your appetite by helping you feel fuller. This way, you eat less, enhancing your fasting.

## 7. Eat wholesome foods during non-fasting days

Non-fasting days are periods full of temptation. You are tempted to eat so much, more than you are used to, most of which are just plain unhealthy food. Some say it is a way of compensating for the days you were not eating. However, this is not the right thing to do in so many ways. First, it does not help create a calorie deficit that is required for you to lose weight. Secondly, it fills your body with toxins that will need excretion in the next fast. Some of these toxins might fail to be excreted as expected. Therefore you end up with a buildup of toxins, and your ultimate goal of detoxification is not achieved. It is, therefore advisable that in between periods of fasting, you eat healthy foods. Eat whole-grain foods and raw vegetables as much as you can. They not only help you feel fuller but also contain components that could help you with your detoxification journey. Besides, they contain nutrients that help boost your energy levels while improving your cognitive functions such as memory, concentration, and learning.

## 8. Keep a journal

It by far the most important of all. If you are into technology, you could use your phone, or you could go to the old school and write an actual diary. Start by writing down your expectations of the fast so that as you progress, you can be able to assess whether or not you are achieving them. If you plan to lose weight, ensure you write down your initial weight. If you plan on attaining glycemic control, ensure you record your sugar levels from before the fast. From the moment you begin your fast, you should write down what time it started and what time it is expected to end. During the fasting period, be sure to note down your progress. How did your body respond? How were your moods during that period of lack? It will help you assess whether or not fasting is suitable for you and how well it is working for you. You could also include photos in your journal as it serves a great reminder of how you were feeling at that specific moment.

## 9. Give it time

Fasting does not provide you with results instantly as some diet loss pills claim. It will take time. Time for your body to adapt to the new system. Time for your brain to know that things are changing and actually to take charge of the new change. For many, it may take as much as several months before they notice any changes. For some, it could take as little as a month for changes to occur. What is important is that you understand it takes time and that everyone is different. Therefore, do not give up if it is not working within the first three weeks. Your breakthrough could be around the corner.

## What to Consider During Fasting

You have already chosen a fasting regimen for yourself and also know to make your fasting successful. That's one step closer to fasting and realizing the potential benefits it as to offer. Before you start fasting here are a few things you should put into mind;-

### 1. Fasting is not for everyone

You may have a friend who has been fasting for the past few months and has realized its benefits. So you now want also to fast since it has worked for your friend, why not you. You need to consider that people are different thus will respond differently to fasting. Furthermore, not everyone is fit for fasting. Some people with some health conditions do not qualify for

91

fasting, and if they do fast, it will be under the strict supervision of a health care provider. These include people with diabetes type 2, heart diseases, autoimmune diseases, or chronic fatigue syndromes. It may also not be favorable for persons under immense amounts of pressure or those undergoing intense physical training. Besides, people who have insomnia may find it difficult adapting to this lifestyle, thus not suitable for them. Teenagers and those over 65 years of age are also not favorable to begin the fasting routine. Therefore, if you are sure fasting is the way to go for you, ensure you check with your health care provider or nutritionist before you commence.

## 2. You need to plan beforehand

You do not just wake up one morning and decide that I want to start fasting. You will need to toy with the idea first, joke about it with your friends, talk to your spouse or children about it, and then consult your health care provider. You will need to make the necessary arrangements to ensure you provide yourself with a favorable fasting environment. You do not need someone continually reminding you that it might not work. You will need to cut such people off. Next is your choice of food in stock in the house. The last thing you need is to complete fasting, and the only thing available for eating in the house is biscuits and cake. You will need to stock up your home or even office with healthier food choices, including fresh green vegetables, whole-grain foods, and lean protein foods. You might need to but yourself a timer or set your phone to remind you of when the fasting starts and ends. Don't forget to get yourself a journal to ensure you do not miss out on recording anything. In simple terms, make a list of what you think you require to make your fasting journey successful and ensure you get each one of it.

## 3. Set reasonable goals

Someone once said that what disappoints us the most is our expectations. As you begin your journey, start by writing down what you expect to gain from this choice you have made. But make sure that they are reasonable and can be achieved. Don't expect to lose all that excess fat within a month. It may take longer or may need to add on another program to be able to achieve your goals. Be smart when setting your objectives to avoid disappointments and frustrations.

93

Think them through carefully and be sure that is what you want to make. It avoids a situation whereby you lose your 60 pounds and look slimmer, but then you realize that is not the look you wanted to achieve. Now you want to put on weight again. Also, we must appreciate that our bodies change over time or depending on our health. Fasting can be working for you great one time, then all of a sudden, it stops working for no apparent reason. You will need to appreciate this and know when to stop when it is no longer working for you and when to maintain the lifestyle.

## 4. Always ensure you meet your body's demands

Fasting fanatics swear that during fasting, they experience heightened clarity and energy on top of the weight loss. It is after the transition period, where they feel irritable, mood less, and have low power to perform even simple tasks. Most people do get to this level. However, you may find it challenging to transition even 7 to 14 days after the beginning of your regimen. It is very normal. It simply means your body is not only finding it difficult to adjust but also that this is not for you. You should, therefore, go ahead and find another suitable method for you to lose weight. Do not insist on fasting, if it is not working for you, as it could have long term detrimental effects on your body. Some may even go into a coma as a consequence of the hypoglycemia they experience during fasting. Therefore, if you still feel light-headed, tired, nauseated, muscle weakness or even faint while or fasting, it could be a sign that it is not what works for you.

It is always important to remember that fasting does not mean starving yourself to death. You still get to eat, though only at chosen times and while following a strict diet. Chose the regimen that works best for you and always ensured you listen to what your body is telling you concerning the fasting. Give it time for it to work, and do not be disappointed if it does not. It simply means your body is different and requires a different technique to lose weight.

# CHAPTER:-7

## AUTOPHAGY AND WATER FASTING

Autophagy and water fasting are two critical aspects that substantially correlate to each other and must be addressed. Importantly, it is essential to understand that most of the body activities which is associated with autophagy are substantially dependent on the water fasting. Other than directly being correlated to autophagy, water fasting increases the rate of weight loss since water is not only a crucial aspect of the body, which ensures normal body operations are conducted but also other substances. This chapter will address water fasting in the broader context, its relationship with autophagy as well as weight loss. It is vital to note that a more significant percentage of the body is composed of water and other nutrient and, thus, whenever the amount of such nutrients is altered, various reactions are observed, especially signs of deficiencies. The body is not only dependent on water, and thus depriving it of other vital substances is a significant harm. To ensure that various complexities such as autophagy are not observed, consuming the appropriate amount of nutrients and water is thus necessary.

## Water Fasting

To understand how water fasting works, it is vital to understand its meaning at first and ensure that any aspect regarding it is also recognized as well. Water fasting thus refers to a period within which an individual takes no form of food but purely drinks water. On stating that a person drinks water, it does not necessarily mean that they take food which contains some amount of water, but they exclusively drink water. Therefore, to assume that you are water fasting, it is your essential role to ensure that you avoid any form of food and purely rely on water. Individuals opt to take water fasting to be religiously based, while others strongly believe it is a measure to reduce body weight.

However, to ensure that you successfully carry out water fasting, it is your role to properly prepare yourself, and it is appropriate to choose a particular time when the body does not require too much energy to avoid various complications. Importantly, there is no accurate time that is put in place under which a person should water fast. However, it is also essential to understand that in terms of medication, the appropriate time through which an individual can go without food is approximately one to three days. Past the stipulated days, a person would be going various complications, which is not appropriate for standard body mechanism. Initially, water fast was generated for religious purposes, but in the natural world, it is principally applied as a crucial factor in natural health, among other aspects.

## Process of Water Fasting

Water fasting may sound to be so much simpler, but this does not necessarily mean it is a natural process; it involves continuous body starving. Anyone taking part in water fast should necessarily note that under no circumstance, they consume any meal and also ensure at least two liters of water are consumed daily. Consuming two to three liters is important since an individual would not get a similar amount of water that they use to get in the meals that they consume. In any case, it is not your first time in fasting, and it is appropriate to accurately plan yourself by lowering the amount of energy consumed, which would further limit you from extreme starvation.

Additionally, before an individual engages in the water fast, it is also appropriate to ensure that food consumption is extremely minimized such that it is easy to adapt to the water fasting process. It is important to note that whenever an individual takes part in water fasting, they are likely to suffer both disadvantages and advantages depending on to what extent it is carried out. There is an intensive process that must be followed to ensure that the water fasting process becomes effective. The process is intensively based on various steps that must be followed one after another.

Following the stipulated steps is critical since they adequately determine to what extent an individual is likely to lose weight. Also, assumptions regarding the steps are likely to result in various complexities that should thus be avoided. It is thus the essential role of the individual taking part in the fasting process to avoid any form of negligence. The following are the steps of water fasting.

## Planning

The first step regarding water fasting involves appropriate planning. Planning is important since it not only assist you in preventing various complexities but ensures that the main goal is achieved. In the planning process, one of the essential aspects to take care of is medication. Any individual under medication should ensure that they don't take part in water fasting. Medications essentially require a lot of nutrients, which would thus be avoided during the water fasting process. Also, there are various medications which when not considered and are likely to be affected during the process. Also, an individual under alcoholism should ensure that at no cost they take part in water fasting since alcohol consumes a lot of water from the body, and when fasting takes place, an individual is likely to be affected health-wise.

It is also in the planning phase that you should ensure that you accurately determine the length that you will take while water fasting. Whenever it is your first time to take part in water fasting, it is thus appropriate that you limit yourself to one day or two days to ensure that the body is not exposed to excessive starvation. In most cases, those individuals who take part in first time water fast and goes for more than two days are likely to suffer from various complications such as excessive loss in body weight as well as other diseases associated with food starvation. Periodical fasting is thus appropriate for individuals who take part in first time water fast other than necessarily making it too continuous.

Also, while planning how to fast, ensure that you consider appropriate time. Determination of appropriate time is likely to be influenced by various factors. One factor, which must be essentially be taken care of is the aspect of stress. Water fasting is appropriate in cases where an individual suffers less or no stress. Taking part in the water fast during stressful times is not recommended since it is likely to impact body operations. Stress not only influences the normal body operations but also lowers the concentration of an individual, which is likely to affect the fasting process. Considering the appropriate time also enables various individuals to prepare for the water fasting process mentally. Mental preparation is effective since it not only prevents individuals from suffering from excessive loss in body weight but also autophagy. It is thus important to understand the planning phase is an essential step in the water fasting process since it determines the success or failure of an individual in the fasting process. Therefore before taking in the water fasting process, it is important to understand that the first step is accurately taken care of. Other making the fasting process effective, the fasting process also prevents any type of complexity, which is likely to be observed during the process.

## The Accomplishment of Water Fast

After you have effectively plan for the water fast, the second phase involves taking part in the fast itself. In accomplishing the aspect of water fast, you need to take between nine to thirteen glasses in one day. Using the glasses is appropriate since it helps you to consume more water than taking directly from any source. However, such an amount of water is also determined by sex, and men should consume nine glasses while men should adhere to thirteen glasses. The difference in sex and water fasting has associated with masculinity among men and not women.

It is also crucial to note that most of the activities which men take part in are purely different from those of women, and thus they are allowed to consume such amount of water during the fasting process. There are various precautions that individuals should take note of to ensure that the water fasting process becomes successful. One of the immediate precautions is to limit consuming too much water at once. Such consumption would essentially lead to various scenarios, such as failing to engage in the process accurately. You should thus spread out water consumed inappropriate manner to avoid any complication. The second precaution involves ensuring that the limit is not exceeded. In other words, under no circumstance should an individual consume more than 13 glasses in a day. Too much consumption of water would also lead to various aspects of hydration which would further lead to failure of the overall process. Excessive consumption of water is also detrimental and would make the process ineffective since there would cause an imbalance of salts as well as minerals.

Importantly during the accomplishment of the water fasting process, you should also combat hunger. Combating hunger, in this case, refers to fighting the hunger itself. Fighting hunger, in this case, refers to the idea of ensuring that whenever you feel you are hungry, you take a glass or two glasses of water. The two glasses would not necessarily fight hunger but would ensure that under no circumstance, you continuously suffer from such aspects of hunger. Consuming water while you feel hungry will also ensure that you do not suffer from various complexities, such as dehydration. One good aspect of taking water while you feel hungry is that it also reduces instances which are caused by dehydration, such as an excessive craving for food.

Importantly, it is also important to note that as you consume such water to combat hunger, they are also among the thirteen glasses for men and nine glasses for women. Under no circumstance should you differentiate such types of glasses? It is thus important to consider every aspect during this stage. Lastly, while in this phase, you should make sure that you totally avoid various cases of high fatty diet since they would directly prevent an individual from achieving various objectives. It is important to note that the main objective of water fasting to reduce a given amount of weight of which consuming some amount of high fat would be contrary to the principal objective.

## Maintenance of Safety During Fasting

This is the last and the most critical step during a water fast since it adequately determines to what extent an individual's objective regarding the fasting is maintained. This step is also important since it determines to what extent an individual can water fast. Water fasting is not determined by how it begins but how it ends, making this step a very crucial step. It is also important to understand that the step also ensures that any complexity which is associated with the process before it ends, such as safety issues are adequately addressed.

In the maintenance of safety, it is thus crucial to ensure that you visit your doctor. This can occur before or during the fasting process. The doctor or the health provider is important since they ensure that safety measures and the client are not affected in any manner. Safety is not only important in reducing negative consequences, which are likely to be experienced but also ensures that an individual is comfortable with the process and can take part in it one more time.

Consequently, other than maintenance of safety through visiting the doctor, it is also appropriate for an individual to be under strict supervision by a trained professional since they can be important in resolving various issues. Fasting under the input of a well-trained person is important since there are numerous requirements that every individual who is water fasting should accurately adhere to. It is thus your essential role to ensure that you identify one trained personnel who will adequately take you through the fasting process to avoid any complexity.

## Relationship Between Water Fasting and Autophagy

As noticed in other chapters, it is important to understand autophagy is a crucial aspect that has not only various advantages but also numerous disadvantages. Autophagy can be related to normal life situations as there are some cases where the car owners opt not to change the whole car but just the battery. Autophagy works in this direction and thus makes body operations run smooth. Autophagy and water fasting are two critical aspects that essentially correlate to each other and must thus be addressed together. It is vital to note that a larger percentage of the body is composed of water and another nutrient, and thus whenever the amount of such nutrients is altered, various reactions are observed especially signs of deficiencies. The body is not only dependent on water alone, and thus depriving it of other important substances is major harm. To ensure that various complexities such as autophagy are not observed, consuming the appropriate amount of nutrients and water is thus important. Importantly, other than directly being correlated to autophagy, water fasting ensures that there are no cases or any complexities, such as various body diseases.

## Relationship between Water Fasting and Weight Loss

107

Other than being related to autophagy, water fasting is also directly related to weight loss. It is important to understand that weight loss is a process that involves the change in the weight of an individual, especially due to a lack of nutrients. Therefore, since water fasting involves depriving an individual self of consuming nutrients, it thus reduces various instances of an individual improving the weight. The body is totally dependent on the nutrients, and thus, failure to consume nutrients reduces the growth rate and eventually loss in the weight. These are the reasons why most of the individuals directly take part in the water fasting to ensure that under no circumstance, they suffer from various complexities, especially obesity and others.

It is vital to note that there is no accurate time that is put in place under which a person should water fast. However, it is also important to understand that in terms of medication, the appropriate time through which an individual can go without food is approximately one to three days; such requirements are important since they directly lower the body weight and not other medical problems. Fasting, whenever an individual is sick, is critical since it lowers body operations. Past the stipulated days, a person would be going through various complications, which is not appropriate for normal body mechanisms. Initially, water fast was generated for religious purposes, but in the common world, it is essentially applied as a crucial factor in natural health, among other aspects. The natural health aspect is essentially the loss of body weight. Water fasting also ensures that there are no cases where an individual suffers from most diseases as the weight is intensively reduced, thus leading to a healthier life.

# CHAPTER:-8

## AUTOPHAGY AND AGING

The process of autophagy and its role in health and diseases has grown high for the past years. Autophagy keeps your body cells in proper balance as it breaks down the cells in your body to recycle them into new cells. Autophagy is also encouraged to yield amino acids that are notelongatedcontemporary to maintain cellular function. If there are disorders that disrupt the normal process of autography, it may lead to chronic illness.

Autophagy drones along with low maintenance level when your cells are receiving what they want in relationto the nutrients that propel energy invention. Nevertheless, when effects aren't working on so well, and nutrient deficiencies strain your cells, viral intruders, and fading subcellular mechanismsautophagy increases at that time and help clear out the infected cells, underperformers, and toxic cells. This helpsguards the rest of your good physical shape cells from harm, which in turn can assistelongatelife expectancy and unhurried the aging procedure and cutting out the risky diseases. The outcome of efficientlyconsecutively autophagy is a cell that is less jumbled with spoiledportions and surplus, and thus a cell that sourcesfewermatters to the matter it is a part of. The stripping of parts and restoring them goes on continuously exclusive your cells at fluctuating charges.

You should be aware that aging moderates the autophagy progression and that gene appearance in diverse species shows a deterioration in autophagy over a period. The gene action indicates that autophagy initiation can be castoff as a policy to encouragedurability. The development of several age-linked diseases like cancer and neurodegenerative ailments has been linked by genetic and age-linkedharm of autophagy and lysosome purpose. Autophagy can also entail essential roles in specific cells of the strength. Both aging and autophagy have been obsessed withfrontwardenormously by the use of hereditarilymanageable model creatures.

Autophagy can as well increase cancer surveillance because it protects the tumor cells once they are recognized in the body and increasing the elimination of aging cells in the body, thus improving your lifespan, it also minimizes your risk to diseases and promotes your ability to age. However, it is appealing to many individuals due to the anti-aging belongings and the amplified metabolic effect that active autophagy leads to numerous health reimbursementstogether with the stoppage of cancer and homeostatic belongings in the nervous scheme. You should know that autophagy is always everywhere. There are three types of autography:

## 1. Macro autophagy

This is just similar to autophagy as it keeps your body cells in proper balance and breaks down the cells in your body to recycle them into new cells. Resources to be cracked down are immersed in an autophagosome, which then journeys to the lysosome and rages with it.

## 2. Micro autophagy

It overwhelms and damages severaldiverseconstructions in the cell; the only alteration is that it draws the cellular contents in the body and then recycles the contents into amino acids for reuse. The lysosome engulfs materials directly.

## 3. Chaperone mediated autophagy

This method targets the proteins explicitly in the body to be degraded. The proteins are then recycled into amino acids for reuse. Very choosy chaperone proteins choice up additional molecules and transport them in the lysosomes. In all situations, the lysosome is at the conclusion of the expedition, where a combination of enzymes will share up the excessconstituents into portionsappropriate for reprocess.

Autophagy is mainly stimulated to take part in the group of amino acids, the amino acids then offervigorover gluconeogenesis since carbohydrates are not readily available and low carbohydrates intake removes the body of easy to access sugars. It also involves the recycling of sequestration and transportation of intracellular materials to the lysosome for degradation.

113

The dysfunctional genes have connected the ailmentsassociatedwiththe irregularmeaning of autophagy in the physique in the body, and the related disorders include:

## 1. Cancer

It is dissimilar from the supplementary diseases in autophagy as it is not hereditarilyassociated but has confirmedreimbursements and dangerslinked with it. Autophagy has cell-protective possessions that stop cancer from establishing, and after a tumor has been recognized, autophagy helps to keep the disease from being destroyed by a standard process to enable your body to fight cancer. However, the cancer therapists are aiming the reserve of autophagy in their patients, which would eliminate the cancerdefensivepossessions, which are thought to have been recognized in cancer by autophagy.

## Parkinson's disease.

The related gene is alleged to sourcechoosydeprivation of mitochondria, which is a cellular construction related to the group of vigor by autophagy, normally known as mycophagy. Parkinson's illness is, however, a neurodegenerative ailment, and it is exaggeratedcontrarily from other complaints.

## 2. Vici syndrome

It is a liberal neurodegenerative complaint that is retreating, suggesting that both the parents need to have it to authorize the gene on the kid to have the disease. The gene-relateddistresses how autophagosomessettled and are tarnished.

## 3. Crohn's disease

It is an inflammatory bowel disorder making it different from the other listed disorders. It is still uncertain if Crohn'sillness is an autophagy-related illness and whether the autography tested rehabilitations would be possible to the handlingchoices since there are numerous genes acknowledged to disturb autophagy; nevertheless, these similar genes are also correlated to numerous other developments.

## 4. Motionless Encephalopathy of Infant with Neurodegeneration in Adulthood (SENDA)

Due to autophagy dysfunction, this was the initial neurodegenerative ailment to be recognized. The gene associated with SENDA affects the formation of autophagosomes, and autophagy dysfunction recounts to the buildup of intelligence iron, which has not been strongminded. This convertedsignificant in detecting autophagy's part in the possible to pleasure other neurodegenerative illnesses with autophagy embattledtreatments.

## 5. Hereditary spastic Paraparesis

This is an alternativedeclining gene syndrome that is neurodegenerative as it affects the lower limbs. It is identified that it impairs the formation of autophagosomes as well as damages the fusion of the autophagosome with the lysosome. However, the role played by autophagy in this disorder is not well understood.

# Hallmarks of Aging in Perspective to Autophagy

## 1. Stem cell exhaustion

Autophagy is essential for the prevention and stillness of hematopoietic stem cells as it is essential to upholdstemness in the bone marrow known as mesenchymal stem cells. As youget old, stem cell actioncuts; therefore, self-renewal is vital to keep the populace of tissue-specific stem cells all overa lifespan. You should also know that forfeiture in elderly muscle stem cells of transgenic mice causes reformedmycophagy all topographies of senescence that reduce the reformativepossible of aged cable cells.

## 2. Deregulated nutrient sensing

Autophagy links metabolic trails to preserve homeostasis beneath a variety of situations as an essential methodmodifying the overall cellular position since autophagy is a catabolic mechanism rumored to be concerned in the cellular and universalbreakdown. Due to a decline in autophagy activity, metabolic strainreplies could be negotiated. After nutrient and growth deprivation are activated and numerous glycolytic enzymes as well as autophagy proteins, thesebrands it probable to attain metabolites cheers to glucose acceptance. Hyperactivation has been found in numerousailments such as foroverweight, metabolic condition, and sort2 diabetes, which highpoints the rank of the constricteddirective of autophagy as well as the nutrient-sensing trail.

## 3. Telomere attrition

117

In favor of the hypothesis, autophagy plays a vital role in suppressing the tumor by an inflection of telomerase movement in the somatic cells. To avoid genome instability and telomere dysfunction, the autophagy response arises, leading to cell survival. Telomerase activity can be reduced after autophagy induction; however, the telomerase movement can care for cell cycle evolution by averting the seizure due to short telomeres leading to reputedmenace.

## 4. Genomic instability

Several representations have provided valuable dataconcerning genomic uncertainty and itsfitting together with vigorous and pathological aging. Autophagy linked molecules act as a protection of genome firmness both straight and tortuously.

## 5. Loss of Proteostasis

The inequity of proteostasisowing to aging primes to protein accumulation, gathering of misfolded proteins, and cellular dysfunction; thus, proteostasis is among the significant purposes of autophagy in healthy materials. Carboxylation due to oxidative strain is one of the variations that lead to harm of proteostasis. Alteration of this trail could notify the usual cell operational, as well as a variability of ailments and usual cell makeup declination since autophagy is considered one of an essential intracellular homeostatic process. To evade cell demise or dysfunction, several homeostatic devices turn on largely in autophagy.

## 6. Cellular senescence

The kind of autophagy, the preciseminute when it performs, and the dwelling where it happens can describe the anti-senescence part of autophagy. Autophagy can meditate the changeover to a senescent phenotype, making it possible to remodel the protein desired to create the senescent phenotype beneath oncogene initiation as it controls the senescence of vascular flat muscle cells.

## 7. Mitochondrial dysfunction

Mitophagy is not only required to eliminate the spoiled mitochondria but also to encourage the biosynthesis of original ones backing up the mitochondrial superiorityregulator since it is the basal procedureintricated in the autophagy deprivation of mitochondria. Mitophagy plays a vital role in cell homeostasis, assumed that mitochondria are concerned in bioenergetics; hence, a reduction in mitophagy is detected in aged creatures contributing to the aging of phenotypes.

## 8. Epigenetic alterations

The affiliationamid epigenetic deviations and autophagy wants to be deeply premeditated to recognize the supervisory loop that appears to be tangled in growth and elderly. Organismal replicas, as well as in vitro trainings, high spot the rank of epigenetics through life when taking together into consideration.

## Benefits of autophagy in anti-aging

- Prevents metabolic dysfunction like diabetes and overweight by encouraging cellular health and revenue

- Fights communicableillnesses by eliminating illness-inducing microbes from exclusive the cells defrayal toxins changeablesoreness and assisting to retain immunity healthy.

- Promotes mind health and protects contrary to Alzheimer's, Parkinson's, and dementia by eliminatingdistorted proteins whose accretion is relatedto the expansion of neurological complaints.

- Boosts muscle performance by substitutingworn-out cells or strained by the exercise with original healthy cells.

- Normalizeirritation by enhancing it as wanted to match off pathogens, lessening it as wanted so that the cells do not persistirritatedforever, therebyoverturningenduringirritation.

## Traditionsto Attachthe Anti-Aging Authorityof Autophagy

There are several natural and healthy habits you can help ramp up the process even if autophagy is working on all the periods in your cells. Here are a few ways that can be applied:

- Use autophagy sympatheticcomplements such as omega 3, fish oils, vitamin D, and MCT oil.

- Always do aerobic exercises like authorityambulatory, running, swimming laps as they all strain the body in the right way, and by doing that, it shots up the autophagy heat.

- You need to contract into steady and not extremeirregular fasting, which due in share to the lack of inward nutrients that stress the physique and arouses autophagy regardless of the provisionalnourishing dip.

- Eat additional autophagy warm flavors such as curcumin, ginger, and ginseng they should never miss in your food.

- You should also drink the autophagy, enhancing teas like green tea and ginseng tea as they promote healthy living.

- You need to go deep into autophagy, exciting foods like coconut oil, mushrooms, lentils, green peas, and pomegranates because they are healthy and don't have any effect on the body.

- Use warm and cold as in adiscontinuous sauna or vapor room time with cold baths as together hot and cold strain the cells encouraging autophagy.

- Don't fail to recall to weight upon good excellence sleep in case you wanted one more aim to get your seal this is because autophagy happensthrough sleep, so you need to get your break and let your cells indistinct out the tiredness while you sleep as it is also advisable.

- You can attempt a ketogenic or deficient carb diet by dropping carb consumption as it enables the cells to be enforced to use fat as their fuel, distributing the body into ketosis because it is a change that assistsincrease autophagy in accumulation to assisting with physique fat loss and dropping diabetes danger.

Do you want to increase your lifespan by living a healthy life? All you need are simple practices such as exercising daily and calorie restriction in your diet. You should also visit your healing to mend and converse the known root causing aging, the earlier the treatment, and the many lives can be protected and avoid exposure to strain as it rallies health the procedure known as hormesis this is because cells respond to pressure by cumulating autophagy mostly irrespective of the kind of anxiety.

Contamination, absence of nutrients, warmth, and

cold can all central to improving long term fitness and lengthen lifespan. Autophagy is an essential portion of this result, and in approximate cases, it is anessential part. Animals with deactivated autophagy do not improve the reimbursements to fitness and durabilitygiven by calorie constraint. The calorie limit may upsurge the extreme lifespan by 40% in rats but not in all other species. In the meantime, someone else who has decent autophagy genetics workouts a lot and limits calories that individuals wouldn't want to take drugs at least until they grow.

Five years of added life anticipation would be about the higher limit of what we might suppose as autophagy is involved in every aspect of aging. You are supposed to have bio creators that quantity autophagy action in a person as a goal, and for some individuals with heredities or illnessesdropping autophagy, they could possibly get considerable benefits from upregulating autophagy to childlikeheights. Obese people with type 2 diabetes also need the drugs that upregulate autophagy to healthy levels. Nevertheless, the forthcoming of persuading autophagy to cureillnesses may be hopeful. Beforehand,beginning any regime, you should look up to your doctor to safeguardyour protection and appropriatediet because the health reimbursementsthat come along are undoubtedly well worth partaking.

In particular, using yeast, worms, mice, and flies has brought about broad requirements for autophagy-related genetic factors to increase the lifecycle observed in several longevity models. There are also numerousoriginal and exciting ways appropriate to autophagy and its character in modulating durability. Autophagy can influence aging and health, and thus autophagy inspiration in select matters have benefits and systematic belongings in increasing lifecycle. Considering these devices will be sufficient for the expansion of enlightening human lifespan based on the intonation of autophagy.

The interventions known as longevity models have also helped a lot in increasing lifespan such as reduced food intake without malnutrition has beneficial effects, dropping the actionheights of most important nutrients such as insulin have also helped in extending life in a figure of types, and pharmacological interventions also have extended lifespan that is polyamine spermidine

125

and herbal phenol resveratrol. The endurance models have engrossed on classifying the molecular machineryfacilitatinglifecycleallowance, together with the parts of diversetranscriptinfluences. All the above longevity models necessitate autophagy-related and lysosome genetic factors for lifecycleallowance in many species.

# CHAPTER:-9

## AUTOPHAGY MISTAKES THAT YOU SHOULD AVOID

The world is all craze about autophagy, what with the alluring promises of the many health benefits and life span longevity, which you stand to gain if you embrace the process. In fact, autophagy is now more popular than intermittent fasting, with many health enthusiasts billing the former as a miracle solution for the many health problems the society is grappling with, including the cancer scourge.

Recent years have seen the development of many ways of activating autophagy, however, one of the most effective ways is fasting and restriction of your calorie intake. This method deprives your body of nutrients and exposes it to undue stress thereby triggering off the process of autophagy by forcing your body to recycle old cells.

Although it is impossible to measure autophagy in humans, it is a well-known fact that when your body has low insulin, and amino acids as well as glucose deficiencies, mTOR is greatly suppressed in order to induce the process of autophagy. This process can also be induced by increasing the AMPK in your body.

Autophagy is fairly a new field and many researches are currently underway, however, there are several conclusions which can be safely made including the may ways on what NOT to do while you are trying to achieve autophagy.

## Mistakes of Autophagy

### Not fasting enough

It is common practice to fast for a period of about 3-5 days for your body to trigger off the process of autophagy. However, this varies with individuals, especially with the way you balance your mTOR and AMPK playing a critical role. You should, therefore, consider several factors before adopting a fasting schedule that works best for you, bearing in mind that there is no standard fasting schedule, which anyone can use to achieve autophagy.

In this regard, there is a common assumption when it comes to intermittent fasting that you can fast as little as 12-16 hours for your body to achieve autophagy and kick out any cancerous cells, regenerate diseased and worn-out cells and basically renew your youthfulness. However, this thinking borders on a fallacy. And this is the reason why:

- First, fasting immediately after meals is impossible because your body needs to digest the nutrients you ate before fasting is initiated

- Secondly, the post-absorptive state of your metabolism usually lasts for over 4 hours after each meal

Bearing in mind the above two reasons, it is obvious that you enter the faster state only after 5-6 hours has lapsed without you consuming any food. Before then, you are still in a fed state because your body is still burning the calories you consumed.

For you to achieve significant autophagy, you will need to fast for longer hours of over 24 hours and a period of not lower than 3-5 days.

## Consumption of Fatty coffee to boost autophagy

Although consumption of fats doesn't elevate your insulin levels the same way high carbs and protein do, fats will still raise your mTOR and get you into a fed state.

It is also important to note that ketones, which come as a result of your body burning fats instead of calories, stimulate chaperone-mediated autophagy as well as macro-autophagy in your brain. These processes usually take place as a result of starvation. You can choose to replicate the process by adding some ketone boosting fats to your coffee such as the MCT oil.

However, adding too many calories from these fats will break your fast because mTOR and insulin levels will be raised substantially in your body. You need to, therefore, limit the ketone boosting fats to about 1 teaspoonful per serving.

It is therefore advisable to avoid any calorie intake if you desire to be 100 percent safe and to trigger effective autophagy in your body. The MCT oil you add to your coffee doesn't really play any significant role in autophagy; they only help you to extend your fats for longer periods by giving you the extra energy you need for longer fasting.

## Consuming BCAAs

Consuming pure amino acids, such as Branch Chain Amino acids can stop your autophagy very fast. When you take these BCAAs you risk getting yourself out of ketosis and stopping your autophagy process altogether. Besides, taking BCAAs can result in some neurotransmitter imbalances and well as mood disorders and thus the need to strictly stay away from them.

However, you can only take BCAA when you are engaging in faster workouts in order to stimulate your mTOR and protein synthesis.

## Artificial sweeteners

When you take calorie sweeteners, your insulin

levels are raised substantially through cephalic phase response, a process designed to release insulin in the gut whenever the need arises.

Insulin secretion is also stimulated when your body is exposed to food through sights, smells, thoughts or tastes. The secretion of gastric juices is also triggered via the same process.

So, when you put anything sweet to your mouth, your gut will prepare for the absorption of those nutrients by releasing insulin. This will result in raised insulin levels in your body which is not good for the autophagy process to take place. You should note that high insulin levels in your body hamper the process of autophagy.

## Supplements with calories

You can break your fast pretty fast by consuming a variety of calorie-containing supplements. These supplements also contain a high level of sugars. When you consume a high amount of these supplements it will add up your calorie levels and make your fast quite impossible. This will prove your mission to achieve autophagy futile. You need 5-7 days fast in order to achieve autophagy, anything less than that guarantees almost no results. You need therefore to avoid the consumption of any caloric supplements during your fasting period.

However, there some supplements which are quite safe such as the herbal supplements, including turmeric, berberine, or mushroom complex.

## Mismatch in your circadian sleep rhythms

The autophagy process takes place effectively when you are asleep. This also applies to the growth hormone, which is normally released between 11pm and 2 am in the night.If you desire to maximize your autophagy, then it is wise to always have enough hours of sleep every day. You should also aim at going to bed early and ensuring you have undisturbed sleep during the first hours in order to maximize your body's physical repair which takes place during this duration.

Avoid mismatch in your sleep hours, such as sleeping for more hours on some days while staying awake on some as this will disturb your autophagy process.

## Failing to do extended fasting

You will fail in achieving your autophagy if you fail to extend your fasting for at least an extra day from the standard fasting days. Extending your fat just for a single day is important in keeping your body in the state of low insulin and low mTOR for longer periods even after you break your fast. You should aim at 3-5 day fast each month. In addition, you should fast for an extra 1-2 48-hour fasts per month.

## Fasting for too long and too frequently

Fasting for too much time to achieve too much autophagy is not advisable, as this could result in some side effects. It is important to take breaks from your fast where you feast and nourish your body. You should also adopt shorter but consistent fasts like 48-hour fast for 72-hour fasts, which guarantee no harm to your health.

# BONUS CHAPTER: 1

## WEEK FASTING PLAN

There are a lot of ways of fasting. IF has been on the increase in popularity eating patterns that entails not feeding or where you restrict yourself to eat some kinds of foods for some periods. This kind of fasting has been linked to a variety of some positive health benefits that have included a short-term increase in human growth hormone and changes to the gene countenance. The kind of effects can be associated with endurance and minor risk of illness. And because of this, it is believed that people who fast will lose weight and have a healthier and longer life. If not appropriately done, fasting can be dangerous. There are fasting plans that you are supposed to follow for you to have a safe fasting period.

### 1. Make your fasting times short

There is no solo way to fast; thus, this means fasting time is upon you. Common routines include:

- 5:2 pattern- you are supposed to limit your calorie consumption for two days in a week. It will be 500 calories in a day for women and 600 for gents.

- 6:1 method- it may be similar to the 5:2 process, but the difference is there is a day of reduced-calorie and not two.

- Eat stop eat- this where you have a 24-hour total fast 1 to 2 times a week.

- 16:8 method- in this method, you are allowed to have food in eight hours, and then you fast for 16 hours a day weekly.

A lot of these procedures advise short, fast times of 8-24 hours. Other people will want to undertake much longer fasts of 48 to 72 hours. When you elongate your fasting periods, then you will have more problems that will entail fasting. This can bring about dehydration, change of moods, fainting, being hungry, lack of energy, and being unable to think. The best way to keep these side effects is sticking to shorter fasting time for up to 24 hours, and mostly when you are beginning. You have to keep in mind that when you fast for longer periods, then you are increasing the side effects like being dehydrated, feeling dizzy, and fainting. For you to avoid such risks, then you have to make your fasting periods short.

## 2. When eating eat a small number of foods

Generally, fasting entails removing some food or all foods and drink for some time. You can decide to remove all the foods on fasting days, but some fasting methods such as the 5:2 diet will allow you to eat up to 25% of your calories required daily. In case you want to give fasting a try, then you have to restrict your calories to make sure you consume little amounts on the days you are fasting for you to be safe and not starting it fully. This method can help to control some of the risks that come with fasting as fainting, feeling hungry, and being unfocused. This can also make fasting more bearable because you are likely not to feel hungry. When you feed on little amounts when fasting and not cutting out all foods, this can help you control the dangers of the side effects, thus helping you keeping hunger at bay.

### 3. Stay hydrated

Slight dehydration can make you feel fatigued, have a dry mouth, feel thirsty, or have headaches. Due to this, you are required to take a lot of fluids during fasting. A lot of health professionals will recommend you to use the 8*8 rule. This is where you take eight glasses of fluid daily, to remain hydrated. But still, the amount of fluid you are required to have should be ranging here thought it is individual. 20 to 30% of fluids in your body are from the foods that you eat; thus, when fasting, it is straightforward to be dehydrated. When fasting, you are supposed to drink 8.5 to 13 cups of water in a day. You are also advised to listen to your body because when you are thirsty, you may want to drink more. However, much you may be able to sustain yourself with the fluids from the food you take, you can be dehydrated still when fasting. For you to avoid this, it's advisable to listen to your body and drink when you feel thirsty.

### 4. Go out for walks or meditate

To avoid eating when fasting can be challenging, more so when you are feeling fed up and hungry. The best way or method for you to avoid breaking your fasting period is by keeping yourself busy. You should engage in activities that will make you forget you are angry. The activities should be the ones involving a lot of energy. The best activity you can do is take a walk or meditate. It should be an activity that will calm you down and not strenuous to your body. It should be an activity that will keep your mind engaged. You have a shower, take a book and read, or listen to some podcasts. When you keep yourself busy with the low-intensity activities like walking or meditating, they can assist you in making your fasting days simple.

### 5. Do not breakfast with a feast

You can be tempted to celebrate by eating large amounts of a meal after your fasting period. When you do this after breaking from fasting, then there is a possibility of you feeling bloated or tired. Furthermore, if you want to reduce weight, then feasting can slow down your long-term objectives by holding them down or stumbling your weight loss. This is because your general calorie quota will impact your weight, intake excess calories after fasting will decrease your calorie debit. The good method for you to break from fasting is to continue feeding in a normal way and go back to your consistent feeding routine. When you take a large meal after your fasting day, then you can find yourself feeling tired and bloated. You should get back to your normal feeding plan.

## 6. Should stop fasting if you have any illness

In periods of fasting, you can feel tired, hungry, or irritated. All these are normal except when you feel unwell. For you to be safe, more so when you are new to fasting, you should consider limiting your fasting periods to 24 hours or less, and you should always have a snack in cases where you will feel like fainting or being ill. When you feel you are sick or have issues with your health, then you will be forced to put on hold fasting. When you experience signs like being tired or feeling weak, then you are advised to stop fasting. Such signs will prevent you from doing your daily tasks, and they will make you have unanticipated moods of illness and uneasiness. At first, you may experience some feeling tired or irritated when fasting. When you begin to feel sickly, then you are advised to stop fasting with immediate effect.

### 7. Consume sufficient protein

A lot of people will try fasting as a method to help in losing weight. You should note that being in a calorie deficit can make you lose muscle in accumulation to fat. A way for you to minimize your muscle loss when fasting is to certify that you are feeding on enough protein on the days that you are feeding. When feeding little food on fasting days, then you have to include some protein to give you other advantages that will include handling hunger. Some studies say when you consume 30% of a meal's calories from protein, and then this can suggestively lessen your urge to eat. So, you should be aware that when you eat protein when you are fasting, then it can assist you to offset some of the fasting side effects. When you have enough proteins when you are fasting, this can help you reduce or control muscle loss and maintain your appetite.

### 8. Feed on a lot of whole foods on the days you are not fasting

People who are fasting mainly are doing it to enhance their health. Fasting is all about abstaining

141

from food, and you should be able to maintain a healthy lifestyle during the days that you are not fasting. The healthy diets should involve intake of whole foods that are connected to a big range of health impacts, which include reduced cancer risks, heart illness, and any other chronic diseases. You can maintain a healthy diet by taking whole dishes like fish, meat, eggs, vegetables, fruits, and legumes when you are feeding. When you eat whole foods, days, when you are not fasting, can help you improve your health and keep you fit when you are fasting.

## 9. Contemplate enhancements

When you are fasting regularly, you are possibly going to miss indispensable nutrients. This can be due to regular feeding fewer calories that will make it so difficult to attain your nutritional wants. A lot of people that are keen to follow the weight loss diets will be most likely be deficient in several important nutrients like iron, calcium, and vitamin B12. When you are fasting most of the time, it is advised to take a multivitamin to make you have peace of mind and assist in preventing deficiencies. A lot has been said, and you are supposed to have your nutrients from whole foods. When you fast regularly, there are possibilities of increasing your risks to deficiencies, more so when you are in a calorie shortage. When such happens, you can decide to take a multivitamin.

## 10.  Maintain mild exercise

You can find yourself able to maintain your daily exercise routine when fasting. When you are new or fresh to fasting, then you are supposed to have a low-intensity exercise more so at first. This can help you to have a good plan and management. Low-intensity exercises include walking, not intense yoga, gentle stretching, and some housework. You should always listen to your body, and anytime you are struggling to exercise while fasting, then it is advisable to rest. A lot of people still manage to go for their daily exercises when fasting. You should have gentle exercise when you are new to fasting and check how it goes with you.

Fasting is not meant for everyone; however, much it can be healthy for a lot of people. You are advised to talk to a dietitian first when you have some conditions like being pregnant, breastfeeding, or about to conceive. If you have ever been a victim of an eating disorder, then you are advised not to try fasting.

143

Depending on how fast it can help in boosting your health. You can decide to fast dietary, political, or religious purposes. A known kind of fasting is the intermittent fasting that has cycles between times of feeding and fasting. For you to be healthy when fasting, then you have to make your fasting times short. You should also keep away from intense exercise and avoid dehydration. When you take enough protein and maintain a balanced diet when you are not fasting, then this can mean you have a general health and prosperous fasting.

When you are a vocational person, then you can decide to fast a day before or after the vacation. This can still assist you in preventing an increase in weight and being sick from diabetes. You should also spend some monies for you to have a healthy feeding plan. You can also choose to fast to help you control your feeding habits or to assist you in reducing or losing weight and at times, prevent diabetes. You can use critical thinking to decide on what characters you want to form; when you are fasting, it's very reasonable to feel hungry. And it is also temporary. The times when you are eating, it is wise to hear more of grumbling and to be hungry. This is a normal feeling, and you should ensure that you have a proper feeding healthy diet.

# CONCLUSION

Thank you for making it through to the end of *Autophagy: Discover How to Cleanse your Body, Activate the Metabolism, and Improve your Life with the Intermittent Fasting*. Let us hope that it was informational and able to provide you with all the tools you need to cut down weight. By finishing this book, you will be able to possess the mastery that you seek in dealing with overweight through autophagy and intermittent fasting.

We have gone through the understanding of autophagy and its role in aiding weight loss. This book has offered easy-to-use but very powerful and effective tools and techniques, including intermittent fasting, water fast, and mindfulness as ways to transform your life to increase your happiness. You are now familiar with what autophagy is, and how it can help you and your loved ones to lose weight. You have also learned that autophagy and fasting are not restricted to anyone, as long as you are healthy.

For this book to work for you, it is vital that you encompass all the advice and techniques you have read herein. It may not be in the order that I listed them in this book, but you must use all of them for maximum benefits. You are now aware of the steps you need to take to start your healthy journey. The next thing you would want to do is put in a request for what you want. Believing in what you want and have settled on is important, and you should not allow any doubts to creep in after.

Finally, if you found this book useful in any way, please let me know Your ideas by leaving a short review on Amazon.